BACKACHE

BACKACHE

IAN MACNAB, M.B., F.R.C.S.

Chief, Division of Orthopaedic Surgery

The Wellesley Hospital

and

Associate Professor of Surgery

University of Toronto

Toronto, Canada

THE WILLIAMS & WILKINS CO.
Baltimore

Copyright ©, 1977
THE WILLIAMS & WILKINS COMPANY
428 E. Preston Street
Baltimore, Md. 21202, U.S.A.

Made in the United States of America

Library of Congress Cataloging in Publication Data

Macnab, Ian.
  Backache.

  Includes index.
  1. Backache. I. Title. [DNLM: 1. Backache. WE755 M169b]   RD768.M27   617'.5   76-40458
ISBN 0-683-05353-1

Composed and printed at the
WAVERLY PRESS, INC.
Mt. Royal and Guilford Aves.
Baltimore, Md. 21202, U.S.A.

To Gillian

PREFACE

*"In seeking absolute truth we aim at the unattainable
and must be content with finding broken portions."*
                    SIR WILLIAM OSLER

Low back pain is a remarkably common disability. Hirsch stated that 65% of the Swedish population were affected by low back pain at some time during their working life. Rowe stated that, at Eastman Kodak, back pain was second only to upper respiratory tract infections in reasons for absence from work. In 1967, The National Safety Council reported that 400,000 workers were disabled by back pain each year and, in Ontario, 20,000 claims for disability resulting from backache are received annually by the Workmen's Compensation Board. However, despite its frequency, backache is not a dramatic disease that arouses the scientific curiosity and interest of medical practitioners. Physicians are understandably disenchanted by the frequently obscure etiology of this irksome syndrome and the commonly disappointing response to treatment.

In an attempt to dispel some of the clouds of confusion that obscure the problem, this book has been designed to present a working classification of the common causes of low back pain and to act as a guide to the examination and management of a few commonly seen syndromes.

Some readers may have no intention of entering into the field of spinal surgery. Surgeons in training always find that a surgical textbook is a poor substitute for experience in the operating room. Because of the rapid changes in the minutiae of surgical technique, a textbook is "dated" as soon as it is written and a description of surgical techniques is of little value to the practicing surgeon who must depend on articles published in medical journals to modify the surgical procedures he employs. However, one has to accept the fact that, on occasion, a patient suffering from discogenic backache comes to the end of the road as far as conservative treatment is concerned. His back becomes a malevolent dictator determining what he can do at work and at play. The physician directing treatment must then decide whether surgical intervention is indicated.

In order that he may give intelligent and informed advice to his patients, he must have some knowledge of the operative procedures, including the preoperative investigations that must be undertaken and the factors involved in the postoperative care. The surgeon in training also needs to know the indications for considering operative intervention and, in addition, must have some knowledge of the general principles of operative technique. The practicing surgeon will understandably skip over the descriptions of operative technique but may find value in a detailed description of the preoperative investigation of obscure lesions.

For these reasons, chapters have been devoted to the preoperative evaluation and operative technique of laminectomy and fusion, and space has been given for discussion on that *bête noire* of orthopedic surgeons and neurosurgeons alike, the failure of spinal surgery.

Because this book is designed to discuss only the principles of diagnosis and treatment, it has been illustrated by simple line drawings. No attempt has been undertaken to make this text into an authoritative atlas of clinical syndromes, radiological changes, or operative techniques.

Although diagnosis and treatment are presented with unmitigated dogmatism, it must be remembered that, with the frequent absence of scientific facts, any treaties on the management of back pain must, perforce, be regarded as a philosophy and, moreover, a philosophy that must be modified to fit the needs of the physician's community.

It is almost impossible to acknowledge all the people who have played a role in the preparation of this book and to thank them adequately. To Mr. Philip Newman I owe special thanks for initiating my interest in the problem of low back pain, while I was still a Registrar at the Royal National Orthopaedic Hospital in London, England. The late R. I. Harris made it possible for me to investigate the pathological and mechanical changes associated with disc degeneration, and his contagious enthusiasm encouraged me to study the clinical aspects of the problem in greater depth.

It was with considerable reluctance that I later accepted the offer made by Dr. A. M. W. White to study a group of patients under the care of the Workmen's Compensation Board of Ontario who continued to be disabled by back pain despite all forms of treatment, including only too often, several surgical assaults. I shall be eternally grateful for Bill White's persistent insistence that I should take on this uneviable task because it was from this study that I learned of the vital necessity to know as much about the patient who has the backache as about the backache the patient has. Dr. Allan Walters led the world on his observations on pain syndromes, and it was from him that I learned of the varying and variable relationship of the disability complained of to the pain experienced.

In the preparation of the manuscript I would like to pay my special thanks to Margot McKay for the illustrations, to Kathleen Lipnicki for the photographic prints, and to Miss Jennifer Widger for typing, re-typing, and retyping the script without complaint.

Finally, I would like to express my gratitude to Ms. Sara Finnegan of Williams & Wilkins who patiently and gently guided me through the task of transforming my handwritten notes and sketches into a form more suitable for publication.

I sincerely hope that our combined efforts have produced a text that the reader can use as a basis on which he can build his own philosophy of the management of this common place syndrome.

IAN MACNAB

CONTENTS

xii   Contents

CHAPTER 1

Anatomy

"You will have to learn many tedious
things which you will forget the
moment you have passed your final
examination, but in anatomy it is better
to have learned and lost than never to have
learned at all."

—W. Somerset Maugham

It is a convention observed by most authors of medical texts to start the book with a chapter devoted to the anatomy and embryology of the subject covered. In many instances this is a form of Brownian movement having very little purposive significance. Having skipped through many such essays, with ill-concealed impatience, it was with considerable trepidation that I elected to follow this well established precedent. I have chosen to modify the usual format markedly and have assiduously avoided detailed description of morphology.

The only purpose of this introductory chapter is to remind the readers of anatomical terminology and to correlate the gross anatomical features of the lumbar vertebrae to pathological changes of clinical significance.

We can consider each vertebra as having three functional components: the vertebral bodies, designed to bear weight; the neural arches, designed to protect the neural elements; and the bony processes (spinous and transverse) designed as outriggers to increase the efficiency of muscle action.

The vertebral bodies are connected together by the intervertebral discs and the neural arches are joined by the zygapophysial joints (fig. 1.1).

The discal surface of an adult vertebral body demonstrates on its periphery a ring of cortical bone. This ring, the epiphysial ring, acts as a growth zone in the young and in the adult as an anchoring ring for the attachment of the fibers of the annulus. The hyaline cartilage plate lies within the confines of this ring (fig. 1.2).

The intervertebral discs are complicated structures both anatomically

1

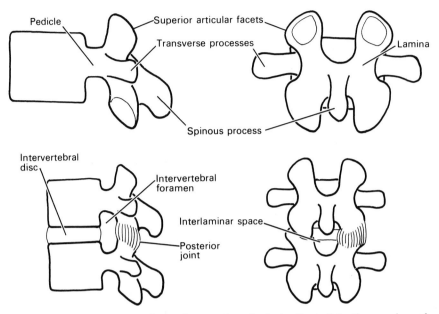

Fig. 1.1. The components of a lumbar vertebra: the body, the pedicle, the superior and inferior facets, the transverse and spinous processes, and the intervertebral foramen and its relationship to the intervertebral disc and the posterior joint.

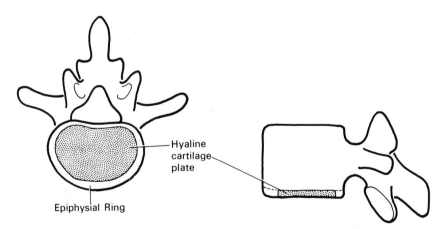

Fig. 1.2. The epiphysial ring is wider anteriorly and surrounds the hyaline cartilaginous plate.

and physiologically. Anatomically they are constructed in a manner similar to a car tire, with a fibrous outer casing, the annulus, containing a gelatinous inner tube, the nucleus pulposus. The fibers of the annulus can be divided into three main groups: the outermost fibers attaching between the vertebral bodies and the undersurface of the epiphysial ring, the middle fibers passing from the epiphysial ring on one vertebral body to the epiphysial ring of the vertebral body below, and the innermost fibers passing from one cartilage plate to the other. The anterior fibers are strengthened by the powerful anterior longitudinal ligament. The posterior longitudinal ligament only affords weak reinforcement. The anterior and middle fibers are most numerous anteriorly and laterally but are deficient posteriorly where most of the fibers are attached to the cartilage plate (fig. 1.3).

With the onset of degenerative changes in the disc, abnormal movements occur between adjacent vertebral bodies. These abnormal

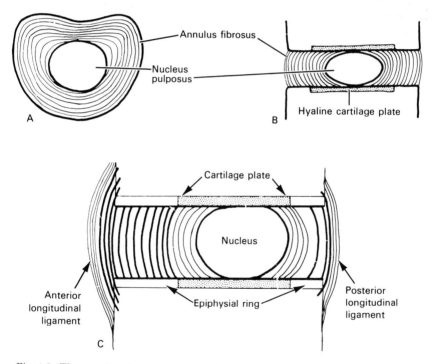

Fig. 1.3. The annulus fibrosus is composed of concentric fibrous rings which surround the nucleus pulposus (A). The nucleus pulposus abuts against the hyaline cartilage plate (B). The outermost annulus fibers are most numerous anteriorly and are attached to the vertebral body immediately deep to the epiphysial ring. The epiphysial fibers run from one epiphysial ring to the other. The cartilaginous fibers run from one cartilage plate to the other cartilage plate. These comprise 90% of the annulus fibers posteriorly.

The anterior fibers of the annulus are strongly reinforced by the powerful anterior longitudinal ligament, but the posterior longitudinal ligament only gives weak reinforcement to the posterior fibers of the annulus.

movements apply a considerable traction strain on the outermost fibers of the annulus, resulting in the development of a spur of bone, the so-called traction spur. Because the outermost fibers attach to the vertebral body beneath the epiphysial ring, this spur develops about 1 mm away from the discal border of the vertebral body and projects horizontally, thus differing in its radiological morphology from the common claw-type osteophyte which develops at the edge of the vertebral body and curves over the outer fibers of the intervertebral disc (fig. 1.4). The clinical significance of a traction spur lies in the fact that it indicates the presence of an unstable vertebral segment.

The first stage of a disc rupture would appear to be detachment of a segment of the hyaline cartilate plate. The integrity of the confining ring of the annulus is then disrupted. Nuclear material can escape between the vertebral body and the displaced portion of the cartilage plate. On occasion, as a result of a compression force, a whole segment of the annulus may be displaced posteriorly, carrying with it the nucleus pulposus and the displaced portion of the hyaline plate (fig. 1.5).

Traction spur

Claw spondylophyte

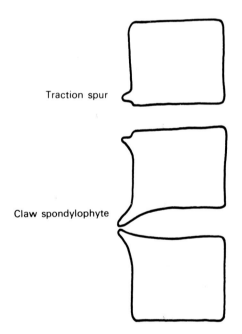

Fig. 1.4. The traction spur projects horizontally from the vertebral body about 1 mm away from the discal border. It is indicative of segmental instability. The common claw spondylophyte, on the other hand, extends from the rim of the vertebral body and curves as it grows around the bulging intervertebral disc. It is associated with disc degeneration. It *does not* represent the radiological manifestation of osteoarthritis.

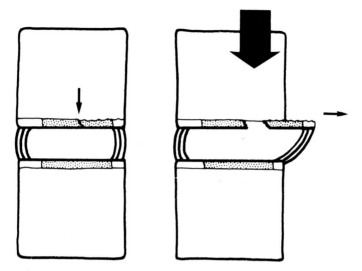

Fig. 1.5. The first morphological change to occur in a disc rupture is a separation of a segment of the cartilage plate from the adjacent vertebral body. Fissures run through the annulus on each side of the detached portion of the cartilage. When a vertical compression force is then applied, the detached portion of the cartilage plate is displaced posteriorly and the nucleus exudes through the torn fibers of the annulus.

The fibers of the annulus are firmly attached to the vertebral bodies and are arranged in lamellae with the fibers of one layer running at an angle to those of the deeper layer. This anatomical arrangement permits the annulus to limit vertebral movements. This important function is reinforced by the investing vertebral ligaments.

Because the nucleus pulposus is gelatinous, the load of axial compression is distributed not only in a vertical direction but radially throughout the nucleus as well. This radial distribution of the vertical load (tangential loading of the disc) is absorbed by the fibers of the annulus (fig. 1.6). This function of the annulus can be compared to the hoops around a barrel (fig. 1.7).

Weight is transmitted to the nucleus through the hyaline cartilage plate. The hyaline cartilage is ideally suited to this function because it is avascular. If weight were transmitted through a vascularized structure, such as bone, the local pressure would shut off blood supply and progressive areas of bone would die. This phenomenon is seen when the cartilage plate presents congenital defects and the nucleus is in direct contact with the spongiosa of bone. The pressure occludes the blood supply, a small zone of bone dies, and the nucleus progressively intrudes into the vertebral body. This phenomenon was first described by

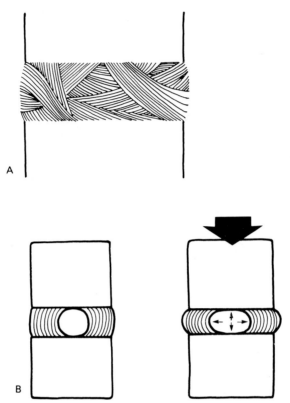

Fig. 1.6. *A*, the annulus is a laminated structure with the fibrous lamellae running obliquely. This disposition of the fibers permits resistance of torsional strains. *B*, the nucleus pulposus is constrained by the fibers of the annulus. When a vertical load is applied to the vertebral column, the force is dissipated radially by the gelatinous nucleus pulposus. Distortion and disruption of the nucleus pulposus are resisted by the annulus.

Professor G. Schmorl and the resulting lesion bears his name, the Schmorl's node.

The annulus acts like a coiled spring, pulling the vertebral bodies together against the elastic resistance of the nucleus pulposus with the result that when a spine is sectioned sagittally the unopposed pull of the annulus makes the nucleus bulge. This has been referred to as "turgor" of the nucleus, but, in actual fact, it is manifestation of a spring-like action, the compressing action, of the annulus fibrosus. This makes for a very good coupling unit, provided that all of the structures remain intact.

The nucleus pulposus acts like a ball bearing and in flexion and extension the vertebral bodies roll over this incompressible gel while the posterior joints guide and steady the movements (fig. 1.8).

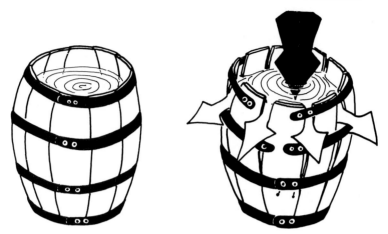

Fig. 1.7. Hoop stress. This diagram shows how the load of water in a barrel is resisted by the hoops around the barrel. When too great a load is applied, the hoops will break. The annulus functions in a manner similar to the hoops around a water barrel.

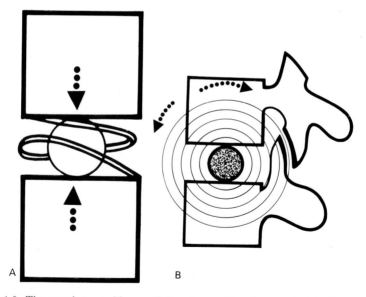

Fig. 1.8. The annulus acts like a coiled spring, pulling the vertebral bodies together against the elastic resistance of the nucleus pulposus. *B*, the nucleus pulposus acts as a ball bearing with the vertebral bodies rolling over this incompressible gel in flexion and extension while the posterior joints guide and steady the movement.

The intervertebral discs have a blood supply up to the age of 8, but thereafter they are dependent for their nutrition on diffusion of tissue. fluids. This fluid transfer is bidirectional from vertebral body to disc and from disc to vertebral body. This ability to transfer fluid from the discs to the adjacent vertebral bodies minimizes the rise in intradiscal pressure on sudden compression loading. This fluid transfer acts like a safety valve and protects the disc. Clinical experience supported by experimental observations has shown that the fibers of the annulus are never ruptured by direct compression loading (fig. 1.9). Sudden severe loading of the spine, however, may produce a rise of fluid pressure within the vertebral body great enough to produce a "bursting" fracture.

Although this has been a very cursory review of the structure and function of the intervertebral disc, it can be seen that the components of a disc act as an integrated whole subserving many functions in addition to being a roller bearing between adjacent vertebral bodies.

The zygapophysial joints are arthrodial joints permitting simple gliding movements. Although the lax capsule of the zygapopysial joints is

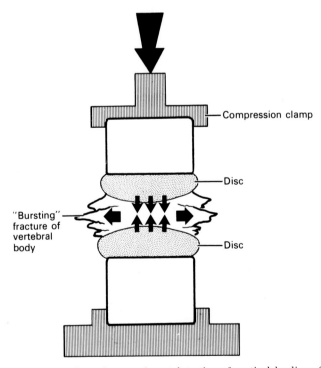

Fig. 1.9. Diagram to show the experimental testing of vertical loading of the spine. When a very high compressive force is applied, the discs will remain intact but the vertebral body shatters.

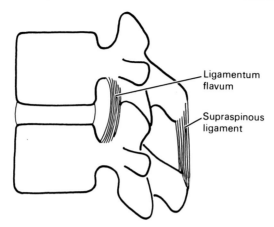

Fig. 1.10. The supraspinous ligament and the ligamentum flavum must be regarded as reinforcing or accessory ligaments for the posterior zygapophysial joints.

reinforced to some extent by the ligamentum flavum anteriorly and the supraspinous ligament posteriorly (fig. 1.10), the major structures restraining movement in these joints are the outermost fibers of the annulus. When these fibers exhibit degenerative changes, excessive joint play is permitted. This is the reason why degenerative changes within the discs render the related posterior joints vulnerable to strain.

One of the important anatomical features of the lumbar spine is the relationship the neural elements bear to the bony skeleton and the intervertebral discs. The spinal cord ends at L1. From this point all of the lumbar, sacral, and coccygeal nerve roots run as distinct entities ensheathed within the dural sac and exit through the lumbar, sacral, and coccygeal intervertebral foramina.

The clinical significance of this anatomical feature is that a tumor can involve any one of the lumbar or sacral nerves at any level in the lumbar spine canal. A tumor may selectively involve the first sacral root at the level of L3 and thereby give rise to considerable confusion in diagnosis.

The nerve roots as they leave the cauda equina course downward and outward crossing an intervertebral disc, passing anterior to the superior articular facet and then hugging the medial aspect of the pedicle before emerging through the intervertebral foramen. At its point of emergence from the foramen, the nerve root is once again in intimate contact with the posterolateral aspect of an intervertebral disc. The nerve root, therefore, is vulnerable to compression by pathological changes occurring at several points during its course down the spinal canal (fig. 1.11).

In this regard variations in the configuration of the spinal canal are of

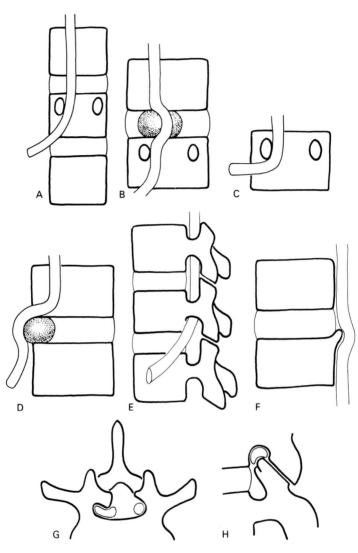

Fig. 1.11. The emerging lumbar nerve roots cross over an intervertebral disc and then sweep around the pedicle before emerging through the intervertebral foramen at which point they are in contact with the lateral aspect of the disc below (A). It can be seen, therefore, that the nerve root can be compressed by a protrusion of the disc that it passes over (B); by kinking around the pedicle (C); and after it has emerged through the foramen by lateral protrusion of an intervertebral disc (D).

In the lateral view it can be seen that the nerve root as it courses down to emerge through the foramen has to pass underneath the superior articular facet and across the dorsal aspect of the vertebral bodies before it emerges through the foramen (E). The nerve root, therefore, may be compressed by an osteophyte derived from the posterior aspect of a vertebral body (F), it may be compressed as it runs through the subarticular gutter (G), and finally it may be compressed in the foramen by the tip of a subluxated superior articular facet (H).

special anatomical interest. The configuration of the normal spinal canal allows ample space for the contained neural elements. However, an anterior convexity of the laminae decreases the size of the spinal canal and a massive development of coronally disposed articular facets decreases the size of the "tunnel" through which the roots must pass to enter the intervertebral foramina (fig. 1.12). In the presence of such anatomical variants, pathological changes in the discs or zygapophysial joints of relatively minor degree may produce root compromise of clinical significance.

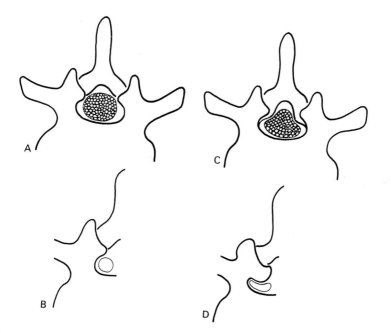

Fig. 1.12. In the normal configuration of the spinal canal (A), there is plenty of room for the cauda equina and the emerging nerve roots course through the subarticular gutter (B) without constraint. In spinal stenosis, the spinal canal assumes a trefoil shape (C) and this anatomical variation not only constricts the cauda equina but also narrows the tunnel through which the nerve roots must pass to enter the intervertebral foramina. When this anatomical variant is associated with hypertrophy of the posterior facets, the emerging nerve roots may be compressed as they pass along the subarticular gutter (D).

Although the lumbar spine is a beautifully constructed multisegmental column, it must be remembered that the necessity for mobility renders it vulnerable to strain. Lucas and Bresler showed that the lumbar spine of a cadaver, dissected free from all muscular attachments, would buckle when placed under a load as small as 5 lb! Morris and his co-workers estimated that when an object was held 14 inches away from the spine the load on the lumbosacral disc was 15 times the weight lifted. Lifting up a 100-lb weight at arms' length theoretically places a 1500-lb load on the lumbosacral disc.

This load must, of course, be dissipated; otherwise the fifth lumbar vertebra would crush. This load is dissipated through the paraspinal muscles and, most importantly of all, by the abdominal cavity, which acts as a hydraulic chamber absorbing and diminishing the load applied.

These observations on the loading of the spine are mentioned solely to emphasize the vulnerability of the spine to the mechanical stresses placed on it by the activities of daily living, particularly in people with poor muscle tone.

Although the sacroiliac joint was regarded for many years as a common source of low back pain, its bony configuration, its limited range of movement, and its powerful ligamentous supports all serve to prevent this articulation from being vulnerable to minor injuries (fig. 1.13). Indeed, it is only when the ligamentous supports of the sacroiliac joint have been relaxed in the latter stages of pregnancy that injurious movements can occur without extreme violence.

Anatomical anomalies of the spinal column are frequently seen. The difficulties attendant upon the diagnosis of low back pain led clinicans in the past to lay the blame for the inexplicable symptoms on diverse and curious anatomical anomalies revealed on x-ray. Although such anatomical variants are legion (fig. 1.14), it has been shown that they do not occur more frequently in the backache population than the population at large and, therefore, cannot be blamed as a source of mechanical insufficiency of the spine. Probably the only anatomical variants that render a spine vulnerable to backache are spondylolysis and spondylolisthesis.

The use, or rather misuse, of descriptive terms of radiological changes as a diagnosis held up our understanding of low back pain for several years. I think that it is a fitting conclusion to this chapter to make the iconoclastic observation that the first question the physician must ask himself, when he has recognized an anatomical abnormality on x-ray, is "I wonder what is the cause of this patient's backache?"

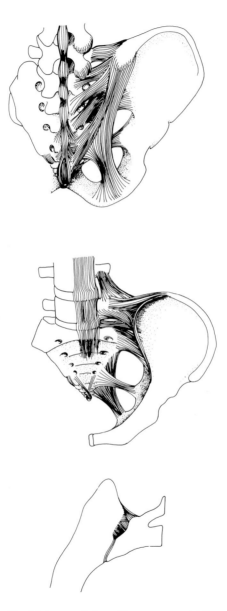

Fig. 1.13. The sacroiliac joints are reinforced by very powerful ligaments both anteriorly and posteriorly in addition to the posterior interosseus ligaments. With this strong ligamentous support, the joint is indeed extremely stable, readily able to withstand the physical trauma associated with the activities of every day living.

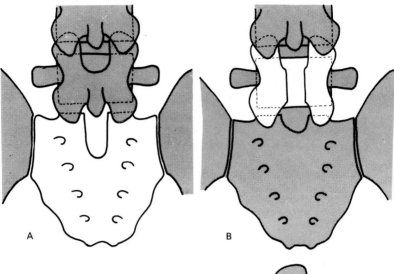

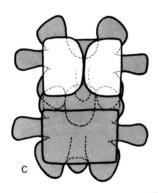

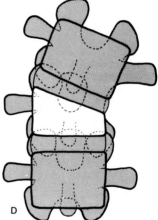

Fig. 1.14 A–D

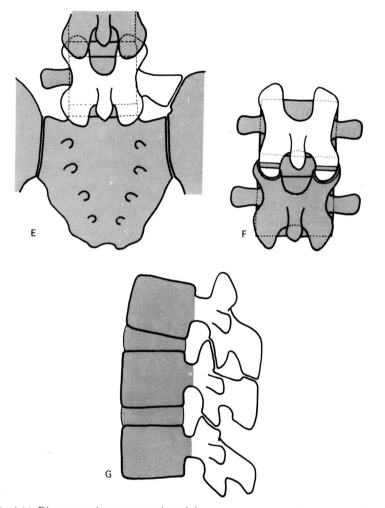

Fig. 1.14. Diagrammatic representation of the x-ray appearance of common anatomical anomalies in the lumbosacral spine: *A*, spina bifida occulta S1. *B*, spina bifida L5. *C*, anterior spina bifida ("butterfly vertebra"). *D*, hemivertebra. *E*, iliotransverse joint. *F*, ossicles of Oppenheimer. These are free ossicles seen at the tip of the inferior articular facets and are usually found at the level of L3. *G*, kissing spinous processes.

CHAPTER 2

A Classification of
Low Back Pain

"Seek facts and classify them and you
will be the workmen of science."
—Nicholas Maurice Arthus

It must be remembered that low back pain is a symptom and not a disease and that the pathological basis of the pain frequently lies outside the spine. The causes are manifold, but may be classified under the following headings: viscerogenic, neurogenic, vascular, psychogenic, and spondylogenic.

VISCEROGENIC BACK PAIN

Viscerogenic back pain may be derived from disorders of the kidneys or the pelvic viscera, from lesions of the lesser sac, and from retroperitoneal tumors. Backache is rarely the sole symptom of visceral disease. Careful questioning will usually elicit other symptoms. The history of a viscerogenic back pain can be differentiated from a back pain derived from disorders of the spinal column by one important feature. The pain is not aggravated by activity, nor is it relieved by rest. Indeed, with severe pain the patient whose symptoms are visceral in origin will writhe around to get relief, whereas the patient suffering from the tortures of a septic discitis will lie perfectly still.

When I was a resident, orthopedic and gynecological outpatients were seen on the same afternoon in clinics on opposite sides of the "great hall." There was a constant stream of patients directed from the orthopedic clinic to seek gynecological opinion as to whether fibroids or retroverted uteri could be the cause of unremitting back complaints. Perhaps it is time that this concept be laid to rest and assume its correct role as a myth or fable of historical interest only. Fibroids and retroverted uteri rarely (perhaps never) cause low back pain.

16

VASCULAR BACK PAIN

Aneurysms or peripheral vascular disease may give rise to backache or symptoms resembling sciatica. Abdominal aneurysms may present as a boring type of deep-seated lumbar pain unrelated to activity. Insufficiency of the superior gluteal artery may give rise to buttock pain of a claudicant character, aggravated by walking, relieved by standing still. The pain may radiate down the leg in sciatic distribution. However, the pain is not precipitated or aggravated by other activities putting a specific stress on the spine such as bending, stooping, lifting, etc.

Intermittent claudication—intermittent pain in the calf—associated with peripheral vascular disease, may on occasion mimic sciatic pain produced by root irritation, but the story of specific aggravation by walking and relief by standing still will make the clinician look for signs of peripheral vascular insufficiency.

The symptoms associated with peripheral vascular disease may be mimicked by spinal stenosis. A patient suffering from this condition frequently complains of pain and weakness in the legs initiated and aggravated by the act of walking a short distance. One distinguishing feature, however, is that in spinal stenosis the pain is not relieved by standing still.

NEUROGENIC BACK PAIN

Although lesions of the central nervous system such as thalamic tumors may present or develop a causalgic type of leg pain, and although arachnoid irritation from any cause and tumors of the spinal dura may produce back pain, the pathological lesions most likely to give rise to confusion in diagnosis are neurofibromata, neurolemmoma, ependymoma, and other cysts and tumors involving the nerve roots in the lumbar spine. The history may be indistinguishable from nerve root pressure due to a disc herniation. Frequently, however, the patients give a history of having to get out of bed at night to walk around in order to obtain relief of their symptoms.

The difficulties that may arise in diagnosis are best exemplified by a patient who presented with severe sciatic pain associated with paresthesia involving the lateral border of the foot and the lateral two toes. His symptoms were aggravated by provocative activity and relieved to some extent by recumbency. Examination revealed an impairment of first sacral root conduction as evidenced by weakness of the plantar flexors of the ankle, a markedly diminished ankle jerk, and diminution of appreciation of pinprick over the lateral border of the foot. His story and findings resembled the classical picture of a herniated lumbosacral disc with first sacral root compression. Myelographic examination was carried out and demonstrated a gross defect opposite the body of L2. At operation, a lipoma involving the first sacral root was found at the point where the root emerged from the conus.

This case emphasizes not only the fact that nerve root tumors can mimic disc herniation, but also the importance of myelography as an essential preoperative investigation in the surgical management of patients apparently suffering from discogenic root compression.

PSYCHOGENIC BACK PAIN

Clouding and confusion of the clinical picture by emotional overtones are very commonly seen. A purely psychogenically induced back pain, however, is not nearly so common. Although the physician must learn to recognize the presence of an emotional breakdown, he must never forget that emotional illnesses do not protect a patient against organic diseases. In such patients, although the task may be difficult, the physician must be prepared to accept the possibility of an underlying significant pathological process and investigate its probability thoroughly.

SPONDYLOGENIC BACK PAIN

Spondylogenic back pain may be defined as pain derived from the spinal column and its associated structures. The pain is aggravated by general and specific activities and is relieved, to some extent, by recumbency.

The pain may be derived from lesions involving the bony components of the spinal column, from changes in the sacroiliac joints; or most commonly, from changes occurring in the soft tissues.

Because these lesions constitute the most common source of low back pain seen in clinical practice, the pathological changes and the pathogenesis of symptoms are discussed in detail in the chapters that follow.

CHAPTER 3

Spondylogenic Back Pain: Osseous Lesions

"The spine is a series of bones running down your back. You sit on one end of it and your head sits on the other."

—Anonymous

Severe pathological processes involving the vertebrae and the intervertebral joints such as infections, neoplasms, and metabolic disorders frequently present as pain in the back. Major trauma resulting in fracture and fracture dislocations may leave back pain as a tiresome sequel. The diagnosis is largely dependent on x-ray findings, and treatment is along well established lines.

Although these lesions constitute a very small percentage of the backaches seen in clinical practice, it is proposed to discuss some aspects of each group very briefly.

TRAUMATIC

Fractures of the transverse processes are notorious for their tendency to leave the patient with a prolonged grumbling low back pain that may markedly interfere with his ability to enjoy himself in his leisure hours. Although the lesions may appear insignificant on x-ray, it must be remembered that fractures of the transverse processes result from gross muscular violence, frequently a resisted rotation strain. The hematoma associated with this gross tearing of muscle attachments tends to progress to dense scar formation, painful when stretched.

The emotionally labile patient who can only proffer radiological evidence of two fractured transverse processes as a reason for prolonged disability may well stand in danger of having his complaints regarded as being solely psychogenically induced, with or without a gain motive.

Persisting pain following a wedge compression fracture of a vertebral body is generally produced by damage to, or malalignment of the related posterior joints (fig. 3.1). If the crush is less than 50% of the vertebral

19

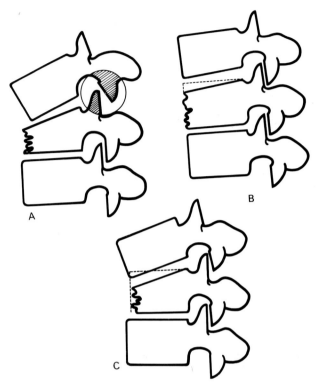

Fig. 3.1. Malalignment of the posterior joints frequently follows crush fractures of the lumbar spine (*A*). If the crushing of the vertebral body is less than 50% the posterior joints can fall into flexion (*B*). If, however, the crushing of the vertebral body is more than 50% of its normal height, then the posterior joints cannot remain congruous (*C*).

body height, the posterior joints can generally compensate. However, if this type of fracture is treated by a hyperextension plaster jacket, all the other posterior joints are held in hyperextension (fig. 3.2). If this grossly unphysiological position is maintained for 4 months, it is scarcely surprising that this iatrogenic damage to the posterior joints subsequently gives rise to prolonged low back pain.

A crush of over 50% inevitably gives rise to a mechanical breakdown of the related posterior joints which will become symptomatic unless spontaneous fusion occurs.

With crushes of less than 50% of the vertebral body height, treatment by early hyperextension exercises generally permits rapid return to full, free function. If the crush is more than 50% the probability of continuing back pain is high. These patients are best managed by a segmental fusion as primary treatment.

The experimental injection of hypertonic saline into the supraspinous ligaments at T12-L1 gives rise to pain referred to the low back, radiating, on occasion, to the buttock and to the greater trochanter (fig. 3.3). Fractures at the lumbodorsal region may also occasionally give rise to low back pain either immediately, or at some time during convalescence. This phenomenon may cause confusion in diagnosis, especially when fractures in this region follow minimal trauma to an osteoporotic spine.

This phenomenon is seen in the so-called "grandma's fracture." Characteristically, grandma goes to visit her grandchildren on Christmas day. They have been given a toboggan and invite her to join them sliding down some steep slopes. Preserving her dignity, she sits on the back of the toboggan with her legs out straight in front of her and her grandchildren between them. As they hurtle down the slope they hit a large bump—the children squeal in delight, grandma squeals in pain. She decides she has had enough tobogganing for the day and elects to go home. Her back is uncomfortable for the rest of the day and when she awakens in the morning she can hardly get out of bed because of *low back pain*.

The pain doesn't clear up after administration of aspirin or application of various liniments. Eventually she seeks the advice of a physician. Various forms of medication are now given, and because these fail to give adequate relief, an x-ray of the affected part, the lower lumbar spine, is

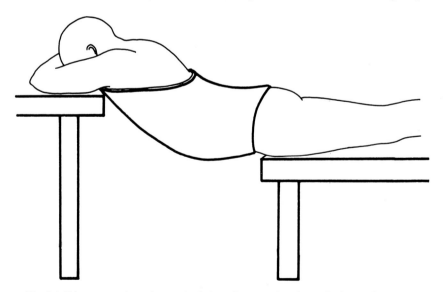

Fig. 3.2. Diagram to show the method of application of a plaster jacket in the treatment of a crush fracture of the lumbar spine.

It must be noted that this jacket holds the lumbar spine in hyperextension.

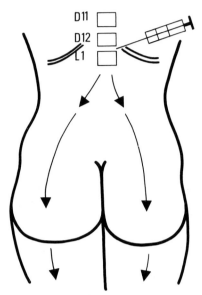

Fig. 3.3. Diagram to show the radiation of pain seen following the injection of the supraspinous ligament between the twelfth thoracic vertebra and the first lumbar vertebra.

taken. This will show a normal lumbar spinal column. Finally, often by error, the x-ray will include D10, D11, and D12 and, much to the surprise of everybody, a crush fracture is seen at the thoracolumbar junction.

This is a very classical example of pain reference. The initial lesion was in the thoracolumbar junction, but the pain was always felt in the lower part of the back. This error, of course, could have been avoided by adequate clinical evaluation initially, where sustained pressure on the lumbodorsal junction would have given rise to local tenderness and probably to pain referred to the lower lumbar spine.

Backache following gross trauma rarely gives rise to confusion in diagnosis. The dramatic precipitating event and the subsequent symptoms are usually indelibly impressed on the patient's mind. The reverse more frequently obtains. It is common for patients to try and remember some traumatic episode and relate this to the onset of their symptoms. When assessing the significance of such a history, it must be remembered that direct blows to the back and falls are extremely rare as etiological factors in persisting backache.

If financial compensation is not at stake, nothing is to be gained by trying to disabuse the patient of the notion that his backache was precipitated by his dog jumping onto his back. The patient is more content to accept such a traumatic etiology and blame his dog than to come to terms with the fact that he's getting older and his discs are degenerating. This may be bad luck for the dog but you are not treating the dog. If, however, the patient ascribes the onset of his backache to a vigorous pat on his back by an erstwhile friend or a blow to the back by the fender of a passing car, then the exact timing of the onset of symptoms becomes of importance. On closer questioning it frequently becomes apparent that there was a delay of several days or even weeks between the traumatic incident and the onset of backache. In such instances and in those patients with a previous history of backache, it is almost impossible to justify the relationship between the injury and the subsequent symptoms. Even in those cases in which the patient insists that the pain originated immediately after the injury, the note made to this effect should carry the rider that the circumstances were most unusual because back pain so rarely follows such an incident.

The exception to this observation is the patient with an osteoporotic spine in whom crush fractures of the vertebra followed very minimal trauma.

INFECTIVE

Spinal infections, despite their relative rarity, must be remembered as a potential source of back pain. For convenience of discussion, infections involving the vertebral column may be considered under the following clinicopathological syndromes: vertebral osteomyelitis—pyogenic, tuberculous, miscellaneous; intervertebral disc "infection," and intervertebral disc "inflammation."

Pyogenic Vertebral Oteomyelitis

Although pyogenic lesions may result from discography, discectomy, and open wounds, hematogenous osteomyelitis follows an arterial or venous route. Probably the most common source of infection is from a pelvic inflammatory lesion with spread occurring through Batson's plexus.

The clinical features of vertebral osteomyelitis have altered from the preantibiotic era. Vertebral osteomyelitis used to be a disease of adolescents and was very acute in onset. The source of the infection was rarely known. Staphylococcus was by far the most common organism involved, and the disease had a dreadful mortality of about 60%.

Vertebral osteomyelitis is now a disease of adults. The onset is insidious and the course is chronic. The source of infection can be localized in about 50% of patients. It is interesting to note that approximately 25% of the patients suffering from this disease are diabetics. Although the Staphylococcus is still the most common infecting organism, Pseudomonas and other Gram-negative organisms are increasing in frequency. The drug subculture has added a new dimension with its own group of Gram-negative organisms.

Commonly two adjacent vertebrae and the intervening disc space are involved. Varying degrees of vertebral body destruction and collapse occur. With the spread of the infection, an abscess may develop and extend either anteriorly or posteriorly. An anterior abscess may spread along myofascial planes and present as a subcutaneous abscess in the region of Petit's triangle or the groin.

Neurological damage may result from the development of an angulatory kyphosis or from a sequestrated disc or bone fragments. Occasionally, the cord may be destroyed by obliteration of its vascular supply.

Clinical Presentation

Backache is the most common presenting symptom; indeed, early in its course the disease is indistinguishable symptomatically from a mechanical backache. The insidious onset and the lack of x-ray changes account for the usual delay of 8 to 10 weeks in diagnosis. With progression of the disease, the back pain increases in intensity, becoming constant, and is particularly noticeable in bed at night time.

All spinal movements and jarring intensify the pain. Paravertebral muscle and hamstring spasms are sometimes severe. It is important to note that fever and constitutional signs are rarely present in the absence of abscess formation.

The findings on examination vary with the stage of the disease. The patient stands with a marked list of the spine to one side. Gross spinal rigidity is a characteristic feature. The spinous processes are usually tender on pressure. The back pain is intensified by percussion of the involved area. Straight leg raising is restricted because of hamstring spasm. Occasionally, a soft tissue mass may be palpated posteriorly or a psoas abscess may be detected on examination of the abdomen or groin.

In half of the patients the white blood count will be within normal limits and even when elevated, rarely rises above 15,000. The sedimentation rate, however, is consistently elevated and is the most useful test for monitoring the disease activity and the efficacy of treatment.

Blood cultures will be positive only if the patient presents with a markedly febrile clinical course.

Radiological evidence of the spinal disease lags 4 weeks or more behind the clinical manifestations. The earliest changes are localized rarefaction of the vertebral end plates followed rapidly by involvement of the adjacent vertebrae and narrowing of the disc spaces. With the increasing recognition of disc degeneration as a source of spondylogenic pain, there is an inherent danger of misinterpretation of the radiological changes. There are no early specific radiological features that distinguish the disc narrowing which is the result of infection from the disc narrowing which is associated with degenerative changes. The radiologist frequently is not provided with enough clinical information, and there is no reason why the minimal radiological changes should make him suspicious of an infective lesion.

At this stage the diagnosis is dependent on the clinical findings: severe pain, a rigid back, and a raised sedimentation rate. Early radiological changes are minimal, but may give an indication of the site of the lesion.

Later in the course of the disease, the x-rays reveal destructive erosion of the contiguous vertebral bodies starting first and usually most extensive anteriorly. Subsequently, there is sclerosis and the development of reactive bone. Evidence of abscess formation is revealed on x-ray by distortion of the psoas shadow or by a localized paravertebral mass.

There may be some difficulty in distinguishing the radiological changes from those produced by a neoplasm, but as a general rule it may be said that with infection the disc space is the first structure to be destroyed, whereas with secondary deposits in the vertebral body the disc space is spared (fig. 3.4).

Treatment

Treatment is dependent on the isolation of the organism and on the stage of the disease. No longer is it safe to presume that the infection is staphylococcal. Because of the increasing incidence of Gram-negative infections and infections by more than one organism, the offending organism must be identified by a vertebral biopsy and culture, in order that its

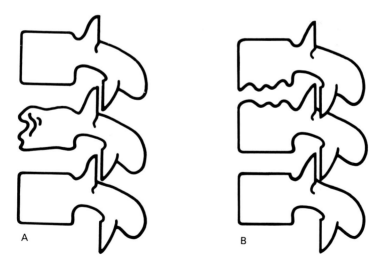

Fig. 3.4. Diagrammatic representation of the changes seen on x-ray with infections of the spine and with neoplasms. With a secondary deposit in a vertebral body, the disc is spared (*A*). With infections the disc is the first structure to be destroyed (*B*).

sensitivity may be determined. If needle biopsy fails to obtain enough material to permit isolation of the organism, then open biopsy is mandatory.

If, after isolation of the organism and the institution of appropriate antibiotic therapy, the patient fails to show any response, the clinician must suspect the accumulation of a large collection of pus. This is not always demonstrated on routine x-rays. A technetium scan, under such circumstances, will frequently indicate the presence of an abscess.

Bed rest should be continued until the sedimentation rate has returned to normal. The patient may then be allowed to get up wearing a well molded plaster jacket in an endeavor to minimize spinal movements. This should be worn for an arbitrary period of 3 months and antibiotic coverage continued over this period of time.

Routine radiological assessment should be carried out at 3-month intervals. Fusion occurs in 50% of pyogenic disc space infections in approximately 1 year, and the majority of the remainder show bony obliteration of the disc space in 2 years. Routine radiological reassessment is of importance because the few patients in whom fusion fails to occur are prone to develop recurrent spinal abscesses.

Tuberculous Vertebral Osteomyelitis

Tuberculous infections of the lumbar spine may present a clinical course that distinguishes them from pyogenic infections. Skeletal tuberculosis is secondary to a focus elsewhere, particularly the pulmonary and urinary tracts. The most frequent site of vertebral involvement is the lower thoracic and upper lumbar region. The vertebral body, as in pyogenic osteomyelitis, in the site of localization. The intervertebral disc is relatively resistant to destruction and simply migrates into the destroyed vertebral body or it may be sequestrated posteriorly.

The disease is very insidious and the time that elapses from the onset of symptoms to admission to hospital may well be over 6 months. In the younger child, irritability and refusal to sit or walk are presenting features. Older children and adults present with simple backache. The symptoms do not have the dramatic disability characteristic of the later stages of a pyogenic vertebral osteomyelitis.

A careful history will reveal the association of constitutional symptoms of intermittent fever, sweats, anorexia, weight loss, and easy fatigability. On examination, marked splinting of the spine can usually be demonstrated. Although the gross tenderness associated with pyogenic osteomyelitis is rarely apparent, localized bony deformity associated with vertebral collapse, presenting as gibbus, is common.

Because of the insidious nature of the disease and the consequent delay in seeking advice, the patient may present with evidence of neurological impairment *even when seen for the first time.*

As in pyogenic lesions, the sedimentation rate is elevated. The white count is variable, however, and may even be depressed. The x-rays do not present any features that distinguish the lesion from pyogenic osteomyelitis. On occasion, an anterior accumulation of pus will produce scalloping of the vertebra similar to that produced by abdominal aneurysms, "aneurysmal erosion" (fig. 3.5).

As noted earlier, tuberculous infections of the lumbar spine are rarely primary. They are commonly secondary to foci either in the lungs or in the genitourinary tract. X-rays of the chest and bacteriological examination of the urine must always be carried out in routine clinical assessment. The Mantoux test, when positive, can be regarded as suggestive but never diagnostic. As with pyogenic vertebral osteomyelitis, vertebral biopsy is essential for diagnosis.

It is possible to treat the patient with antituberculous drugs and immobilization. However, anterior debridement of the lesion with immediate grafting is probably the treatment of choice. Surgical ablation of the tuberculous lesion significantly shortens the course of the disease process, and the incidence of deformity and neurological complications is markedly reduced.

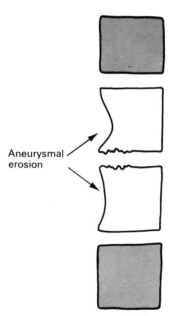

Aneurysmal erosion

Fig. 3.5. When an abscess forms on the anterior surface of the vertebral column, the x-ray shows scalloping of the vertebral bodies.

Because a similar type of scalloping is seen with abdominal aneurysms, this radiological lesion is sometimes referred to as "aneurysmal erosion."

It must be emphasized once again that, unlike pyogenic osteomyelitis, tuberculous lesions of the vertebral column are commonly associated with neurological lesions. In such instances, the prognosis following decompression carried out early is excellent. In contrast, in neglected cases, paraplegia caused by penetration of the dura and involvement of the cord by tuberculous granulation tissue produces irreversible changes.

Miscellaneous Infections of the Spine

Uncommon Pyogenic Lesions

The spine may be involved by typhoid or by brucellosis. Unlike other pyogenic infections, the vertebral body frequently shows a reactive sclerosis appearing like a white block on x-ray.

Fungal

Fungi can establish growth within bony tissue—mycotic osteomyelitis. The most common fungi seen are coccidial mycosis, blastomycosis, and actinomycosis. The skeleton, however, is rarely involved except as part of a disseminated disease. From a clinical standpoint, it must be remembered that each one of these mycotic infections can mimic tuberculosis radiologically, again emphasizing the need for vertebral biopsy as an essential part of establishing the diagnosis and initiating appropriate treatment.

Parasitic

Hydatid disease has been known as a clinical entity from ancient times. When bone involvement is present, the spine is also involved in about 18% of patients. Diagnosis is difficult. X-rays reveal lytic lesions in the vertebral body. Neurological involvement occurs early and relentlessly progresses to an irreversible paraplegia. To date, it would appear that treatment fails to obtain any significant response.

Syphilis

The incidence of syphilitic bone and joint involvement has decreased from 36% in 1900 to less than 0.5% in 1936 and this decline has been maintained. Charcot arthropathy is the most common manifestation of syphilitic involvement of the vertebral column and is seen most frequently at the thoracolumbar junction. Although the lesion may be symptomless and detected solely by incidental x-rays, pain may arise when destructive and hypertrophic changes are marked. Similar changes may be seen with diabetes, although this is rare. Complete collapse of the vertebral column may occur with transection of the cord or cauda equina.

Intervertebral Disc Space Infection

Disc space infections may occur following surgical enucleation of a herniated intervertebal disc. The clinical picture is fairly characteristic. There is an initial relief of the preoperative pain following the discectomy. Approximately 1 to 8 weeks later, severe backache occurs with marked cramps of pain. The pain is described as being "excruciating" and is out of proportion to the objective findings.

There are very few constitutional symptoms except in those patients who run a febrile course. The sedimentation rate is, however, elevated and is useful in following the subsequent treatment program.

X-rays do not show abnormality for about 4 or 6 weeks when for the first time narrowing of the disc space is revealed. This narrowing occurs much earlier than the anticipated narrowing subsequent to the physical act of disectomy and, of course, is much more marked. Later, irregularity and loss of definition of the vertebral end plates are noted with subsequent vertebral destruction. More than half of the patients progress to disc space obliteration and interbody fusion.

Aspiration by needle biopsy is essential to establish a bacteriological diagnosis in order that the lesion may be treated by appropriate antibiotics. The treatment in essence is the same as the treatment of pyogenic vertebral osteomyelitis.

Intervertebral Disc Inflammation

This is a benign condition occurring only in children. Confusion regarding the etiology has resulted in a multitude of synonyms: acute infectious lesions of the intervertebral discs, spondyloarthritis in children, benign acute osteitis of the spine, nonspecific spondylitis, and discitis.

This confusion indicates that as yet the etiology is unknown. Objective data from the literature and personal experience lend support to an infectious etiology; however, until substantiated, the term inflammation is preferred to infection.

In contrast to vertebral osteomyelitis, intervertebral disc inflammation most commonly presents between the ages of 2 and 6. Infants refuse to walk and older children complain of hip or back pain. There are few localizing signs early in the course of the disease. Later typical findings of restricted spinal mobility, paravertebral and hamstring muscle spasm, and pain on percussion over the lumbar spine are present. The children are afebrile on examination.

The single most consistent laboratory finding is the elevated sedimentation rate which may be well over 50. Blood cultures are not positive; indeed, if a positive blood culture is obtained, the condition should no longer be considered an inflammation, but should be regarded as vertebral osteomyelitis and treated as such.

There is a 2- or 4-week delay before x-ray changes are present. The lumbar vertebrae are most commonly involved, especially the fourth lumbar vertebra. The earliest sign is narrowing of a disc space which may be seen to progress for an additional 1 or 2 months. This change may be associated with irregular erosion of the vertebral end plates and, on occasion, the disc may balloon into the vertebral body. However, wedging and vertebral collapse do not occur. Tomography has occasionally demonstrated cavitation in the vertebral body which, interestingly enough, will persist after apparent healing. A bone scan may localize the level of pathology before x-ray changes are apparent.

In the natural history of the disease, the disc height is usually restored and the end plates regain their definition.

The essence of treatment is immobilization. Without any knowledge of the presence and nature of any organisms, the empirical administration of antibiotics is illogical and of debatable value. Systemic signs, fever, leukocytosis, or failure to improve on bed rest are indications for biopsy to differentiate the syndrome of disc space inflammation from vertebral osteomyelitis and in the latter instance to institute appropriate antibiotic therapy.

NEOPLASTIC

The diagnosis of neoplasms of the vertebral column is largely dependent on x-ray examinations. This text is not intended as an atlas of lesions of the vertebral column and no attempt is made here to describe the specific radiological and histological characteristics of the tumors that occur. An attempt is made to outline the principles of diagnosis and treatment.

Benign neoplasms and primary malignancies in the vertebral column are rare. Secondary deposits are common.

Benign Tumors

Benign tumors predominately affect the under 30 generation. Backache, at the site of the lesion, is the dominant symptom, and this may be associated with a painful scoliosis. Idiopathic scoliosis is rarely painful. When a patient presenting with a scoliosis complains of severe backache, remember the possibility of a benign tumor and examine its probability with detailed radiological assessment.

Benign lesions usually occur in the posterior elements or accessory processes and present two specific difficulties in evaluation and treatment. First there is the difficulty in demonstrating the lesion on x-ray. When clinical suspicion is high, but radiological findings are equivocal, then a technetium bone scan is useful. If the scan can localize the tumor and confirm a lesion, tomography may then be employed to further define its exact site and characteristics. When the scan is negative, then plain x-rays and the scan should be repeated after a 3-month interval if the clinical problem persists.

Second, benign lesions may be inaccessible for surgical removal. However, incomplete removal may be all that is necessary.

The following is a summary of the clinical features of the more commonly seen benign lesions.

Hemangioma

Characteristically on x-ray the affected vertebra demonstrates linear striations giving rise to a corduroy cloth or honey-combed appearance (fig. 3.6). This radiological finding can be demonstrated in nearly 12% of all vertebral columns, with the incidence increasing with age. The incidence in the backache population is no greater, emphasizing the fact that the mere demonstration of a hemangioma of a vertebral body on x-ray does not indicate that the source of the patient's backache has been found.

Treatment is simply observation. In a few patients with constant disabling pain, if the symptoms can be reproduced or aggravated by the intraosseous injection of saline into the affected vertebral body and if the pain is completely relieved by recumbency, then a posterior bypass graft, by unloading the affected segment, will alleviate the pain.

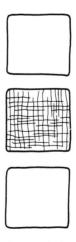

Fig. 3.6. Diagram to show the characteristic x-ray appearance of the so-called hemangioma of the vertebral body. The vertical and horizontal trabeculae are accentuated giving a corduroy cloth or honey-combed appearance.

Medullary Island

These radiologically demonstrated discrete osteosclerotic foci seen on x-rays are composed of normal compact bone. They have no clinical significance, but care must be taken not to confuse them with osteoblastic metastases.

Osteoid Osteoma

The most common clinical presentation is a gradual progressive backache. The majority of the patients (80%) are between 5 and 25 years of age. It can be said that backache in children or young adults associated with marked paravertebral muscle spasm and the sudden onset of scoliosis warrants consideration of an osteoid osteoma. On x-ray the lesion most frequently is seen to involve the accessory, spinous, transverse, or articular processes. Although on occasion symptoms occur before it is possible to demonstrate the lesion on x-ray, typically there is an area of dense sclerosis surrounding a central radiolucent nidus.

The most successful form of treatment is a local excision of the tumor.

Osteoblastoma

In contrast to all other primary neoplasms of bone, osteoblastoma manifests a most distinct predilection for the spine. Forty per cent of all osteoblastomata are found in the spine, almost invariably in the posterior elements of the lumbar spine and sacrum. The tumor is seen most commonly in males and 80% of the patients are under 30 years of age.

Back pain is always the presenting symptom with significant scoliosis being demonstrated in more than half of the cases. Because of the expansile nature of the tumor, many of the patients will present, on examination, some evidence of a neurological deficit.

Treatment is by surgical excision and even incomplete removal is compatible with complete symptomatic relief.

Eosinophilic Granuloma

This is a proliferative disorder of histiocytes. Vertebral involvement presents as a variable degree of compression of a vertebral body without any evidence of an adjacent soft tissue mass. In the extreme form, the vertebra is flattened to a thin disc, so-called vertebra plana (fig. 3.7). This spontaneous collapse of the vertebral body in children was first described by Calvé. It was thought to be a manifestation of osteochondritis juvenilis and is still referred to as "Calve's disease." The lesion responds to low dose radiation therapy and the prognosis is excellent. A word of caution. Any secondary deposit may cause wedging of a vertebral

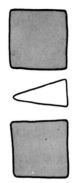

Fig. 3.7. Wedging of the vertebral body associated with Calvé's disease.

body, and this possibility must be considered carefully before making the diagnosis of Calve's disease.

Aneurysmal Bone Cyst

This tumor generally presents as a solitary expansile lesion involving the vertebra. Although the tumor is seen in all age groups, 90% of the patients are under 20 years of age. The clinical presentation is one of back pain with or without neurological symptoms developing as a result of the expansile nature of the tumor.

X-rays reveal a destructive expansile lesion but characteristically the cortex remains intact.

It is the only benign lesion that may extend from one bone to another in the vertebral column.

Treatment is by excision and spinal fusion to restore stability. It is to be noted that operative excision may at times be a horrendously hemorrhagic experience.

Giant Cell Tumors

Fortunately, this is an extremely uncommon tumor of the vertebral column. Although the lesion is not commonly malignant, it is certainly more malevolent than benign, with a greater than 60% recurrence rate following local resection and bone grafting.

Malignant Tumors

Malignant lesions, primary or secondary, are affections of the over 40 population, their incidence increasing with age. The tumors almost invariably involve the anterior spinal elements.

Backache is the presenting symptom, although neurological manifestations may arise not only because of the lesion is expansile, but also from vertebral collapse and direct extradural extension. Early in the natural history of the disease the lesions may not be demonstrated on x-ray. It must be remembered that 30% of the osseous mass of a bone must be destroyed before a lesion is radiologically evident. In autopsy specimens, only 15% of grossly affected vertebrae demonstrated recognizable lesions when the excised spines were x-rayed. When routine x-rays fail to demonstrate any abnormality, a technetium scan can be of value in defining the presence of the lesion and the extent of spinal involvement.

The concept of "disease extent" is critical in the treatment of spinal malignancies. Solitary lesions, primary or metastatic, have a better prognosis for survival and warrant an active search for the primary, with aggressive surgical or radiotherapeutic measures to the secondary lesions.

The laboratory findings, such as alterations in the blood levels of calcium, phosphorus, alkaline and acid phosphatases, and globulins may suggest malignant disease and can on occasion identify entities such as myeloma. Final confirmation of the nature of the lesion may require percutaneous or open biopsy.

Primary Malignant Tumors

Although primary malignant lesions are rare, the following may be seen.

Chordoma. This is a slowly developing, locally invasive and destructive tumor originating from remnants of notochordal tissue with a distinct predilection for either end of the spinal column with a midline localization.

It is uncommon before the age of 30 and is found mostly in males. Interestingly enough, although the tumor is locally aggressive with a 10% incidence of metastases, the symptoms are frequently of long duration. Pain in the lower back, sacrum, and coccyx are early and persistent symptoms. Characteristically, as with all tumors of the spinal column, the pain is not relieved by recumbency. As the tumor encroaches on the sacral foramina, neuropathies and bowel and bladder symptoms appear. Neurological involvement is usually later in the natural history of the tumor.

X-rays reveal a large lytic lesion of the sacrum with a large soft tissue mass almost indistinguishable from the x-ray appearance of a giant cell tumor. However, a chordoma is much more commonly seen in men, whereas giant cell tumors occur with greater frequency in women. A chordoma is not seen until well beyond the third decade, whereas giant cell tumors are more frequently encountered below the age of 30. A giant cell tumor progresses usually more rapidly than a chordoma and unlike a chordoma may be situated away from the midline.

Therapeutically, both lesions present problems. Total excision is the goal of any surgery. Sacral tumors restricted to the lower two or three sacral segments can be removed by a combined abdominal and sacral approach. This excision will leave satisfactory anal and bladder sphincter function.

Myeloma. This is the most common primary malignant tumor of the spine. The disseminated form of myeloma is uncommon below the age of 50 and is more often seen in males. Clinically, backache, weakness, weight loss, and other constitutional symptoms occur in nearly every patient with the generalized disease. The onset of pain may be sudden and is usually produced by the development of a pathological fracture.

The sedimentation rate is consistently elevated and is usually greater than 50. Laboratory investigations may reveal hypercalcemia, hyperurecemia, and an elevation in the alkaline phosphatase. Characteristically, the disease is associated with abnormal proteins. Bence Jones proteinuria may be demonstrated in about 50% of the cases. Generally, when the globulins are normal the albumin is normal. The albumin decreases when the globulins are elevated, reflecting damage to the renal tubules.

On x-ray the solitary lesions are purely lytic and do not show any attempt at regeneration of bone. The disseminated form frequently shows nothing more than a diffuse osteopenia with or without vertebral body crush.

Treatment of solitary lesions is predicated on preservation of spinal stability and cord function. In the absence of gross spinal instability, management with radiation and chemotherapy is probably the best mode of treatment. Spinal instability may require excision of the lesion and bypass grafting.

Cord impairment makes decompression mandatory. Depending on the number of segments affected and the type of encroachment on the cord, decompression may have to be performed either anteriorly or posteriorly. This may seem excessive surgery for a malignant lesion, but is should be remembered that solitary lesions have a 5-year survival rate of about 60%.

Metastatic Tumors

The spine is the most common site of metastatic spread in the skeleton, and the lumbar vertebrae are the most frequently involved. The x-rays of the spine may be normal since 30% of the osseous mass of a bone must be destroyed before a lesion is radiologically apparent. In autopsy specimens, only 15% of grossly affected vertebrae demonstrate recognizable lesions when the excised specimen is x-rayed.

Most lesions in the vertebrae are osteolytic. Markedly osteolytic metastases are seen with hypernephroma, thyroid, and large bowel carcinoma. Breast, prostate, and lung tumors may produce osteoblastic metastases.

Back pain due to spinal metastases may be the presenting finding in about 25% of patients suffering from malignant lesions. Any patient over the age of 50 who presents with the history of low back pain of sudden onset without provocative trauma, unrelieved by rest in bed, associated with sudden cramps of pain, and a significantly elevated sedimentation rate should be suspected of suffering from a secondary deposit in the spine unless proved otherwise. The concern is even greater if the patient has a previous history of a malignant lesion.

The x-rays may be normal or the changes may be minimal indeed. A careful examination of the anteroposterior view of the spine may show the absence of one pedicle, the "winking owl sign" (fig. 3.8).

When destructive lesions of the vertebral bodies are demonstrated, it is important to distinguish between neoplasms and infections. As a general rule, it may be said that the disc space is involved with infections and it is spared with neoplasms. Occasionally, despite a clinical picture that is highly suggestive of secondary deposits in the spine, the only abnormality on x-ray examination is a diffuse osteoporosis of the vertebral column

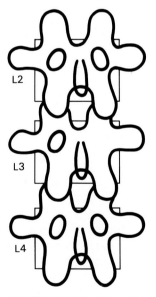

Fig. 3.8. Absence of one pedicle (the third lumbar vertebra depicted in this diagram) is often the first and only sign of a secondary deposit in the lumbar spine.

The x-ray appearance is sometimes referred to as the "winking owl sign."

with or without a minor vertebral body crush. In such a patient, a disciplined use of laboratory findings followed where indicated by a technetium scan and trephine biopsy is necessary to establish the diagnosis and define treatment.

In those patients in whom x-rays show a destructive vertebral lesion irrefutably due to a secondary malignant deposit and in whom there is no evidence of the site of the primary, the question arises as to whether there is any value in carrying out a biopsy. The cell morphology in the secondary deposit is frequently so altered as to make it almost impossible to be more specific than "adenocarcinoma" or "epithelial tumor." In such instances, little has been gained except to assess the radiosensitivity or in the case of a very anaplastic lesion, the prognosis. However, one has to accept the fact that on occasion a specific diagnosis can be made such as an unsuspected myeloma or a lymphoma. Under such circumstances, more specific modes of therapy can be instituted, depending on whether the lesion is hormone-dependent or chemically controllable. The disease in such patients may run a slow course, and in certain instances, the surgeon might be justified in carrying out a biological stabilization with a bone graft.

On the other hand, when the prognosis is extremely grave in a patient whose general health is deteriorating, the debilitating pain can be humanely controlled by grouting the spine with a cold setting plastic reinforced with micrographite fibers. The pain relief obtained by such means can, on occasion, be very gratifying and the procedure, therefore, justifiable despite the unremitting, relentless, and often rapid progress of the lesion.

Over one-quarter of the patients with spinal metastases present with neurological dysfunction. In tumors which frequently run a long clinical course, this is a disasterous complication. The prognosis is related to the following factors: (1) The level of neurological dysfunction. Over 80% of the tumors producing neurological defects occur at the thoracic cord level. The more proximal the level of cord involvement, the poorer the prognosis. (2) Duration of neurological dysfunction. As a rule the longer the signs are present, the worse the prognosis. (3) The onset of neurological signs. The more rapid the onset, the less favorable the prognosis. (4) Sphincter involvement. Sphincter involvement is indicative of an extremely poor prognosis.

It can be said as a generalization that two-thirds of the patients who are operated on for neurological defects can maintain their preoperative status. One-third of those who are unable to walk before operation can once again, for a period of time, get up and get around.

The timing of the decompression is of importance, and it would appear that if a decompression is indicated then it must be carried out as an emergency procedure if any measure of recovery is to be expected. The surgical decompression must be performed with the meticulous technique employed in the decompression of acute traumatic lesions. Careless handling of the cord can convert a partial lesion into a complete lesion.

The management of metastatic spine lesions ranges from the simple to the complex. Experience, personal philosophy, and the patient are at times the only guides to this, the most difficult of orthopedic problems.

METABOLIC

The vertebral column may be involved in any metabolic bone disease such as osteofibrosis, osteopetrosis, alkaptonuria, familial hypophosphatemia, etc. The metabolic bone disease most commonly presenting with the symptom of back pain is osteoporosis. It is proposed therefore to restrict the description of the role of metabolic bone disease in the production of back pain to a discussion of the diagnosis and treatment of primary osteoporosis.

Osteoporosis may be considered as primary or secondary. Primary osteoporosis is classified into very vague groups: idiopathic juvenile osteoporosis, idiopathic osteoporosis of adults, menopausal osteoporosis, and senile osteoporosis.

Idiopathic juvenile osteoporosis is a rare condition affecting children between the ages of 8 and 12. It runs a 2- or 3-year course and then regresses spontaneously. Idiopathic osteoporosis of adults is more common in men. It usually becomes clinically evident at 40 years of age and the symptoms may persist for 5 to 10 years. Postmenopausal and senile osteoporosis are the most common types of primary osteoporosis. The causes of secondary osteoporosis are legion (table 3.1).

Osteoporosis results from an imbalance of bone formation and bone resorption. In postmenopausal and senile osteoporosis, although both formation and resorption of bone are diminished, the rate of resorption exceeds the rate of formation. Many theories have been expounded to explain this curious phenomenon. It has been postulated that estrogen deficiency renders bone more susceptible to the action of parathyroid hormone. Some contend that a high intake of meat in the diet increases hydrogen ion excretion in the urine which is buffered at the expense of bone. Predictably it has been suggested that a long standing calcium deficiency in the diet leads to secondary hyperparathyroidism and bone resorption. None of these theories has been proven. It is, however, of interest to note that osteoporosis rarely occurs in areas where there is a high fluoride content in the drinking water.

The presenting symptom of vertebral osteoporosis is backache. The pain is spondylogenic in nature, being aggravated by general and specific

Table 3.1. A General Classification of Osteoporosis

Regional	Disuse
	Post-traumatic osteodystrophy
	Migratory
	Inflammatory
General	
Congenital	Osteogenesis imperfecta
	Homocystinuria
Acquired	Idiopathic
	Juvenile
	Postmenopausal
	Senile
	Hormonal
	Hyperthyroidism
	Hyperadrenocorticism (endogenous or exogenous)
	Acromegaly
	Hypogonadism
	Neoplastic
	Multiple myeloma, and leukemia
	Bone metastases
	Hormone-producing tumors
	Myeloproliferative
	Sickle cell anemia
	Thalassemia
Compound	Associated with hyperparathyroidism, and some cases of osteomalacia

activities and being relieved to some extent, but not completely, by recumbency.

The pain has been ascribed to trabecular buckling or trabecular fractures. This is an untenable hypothesis when faced with the fact that trephine biopsies of the vertebral bodies can be performed painlessly. When considering the cause of pain, it must be remembered that although the bone mass has been markedly diminished, the size of the vertebral body remains the same. If the quantity of bone has been decreased, then the other contents of the vertebral body must increase: the marrow, the fat and the blood lakes. The fat content of an osteoporotic vertebral body does not increase. Therefore, it must be presumed that the volume of the blood lakes must be greater. This implies venous stasis. The interosseus venous pressure of a normal vertebra is about 28 mm Hg. The interosseus venous pressure of an osteoporotic vertebral body is approximately 40 mm Hg. It is known that intraosseus venous stasis is seen in juxta-articular bone in osteoarthritis and that this is reversed following osteotomy. The decrease in venous pressure following osteotomy and following forage of the hip joint for osteoarthritis probably accounts for the relief of pain experienced in the immediate postoperative period. It is probable that venous stasis in the vertebral bodies plays a significant role in the production of the dull, nagging, constant, boring pain of which these patients so commonly complain.

Although trabecular fractures do not play a role in the reproduction of symptoms, crush fractures of a vertebral body are common and some are associated with the sudden onset of severe pain.

Fractures of the vertebral column are usually first noted in the thoracic region. Involvement of several upper thoracic vertebral bodies over a course of time may produce an increasing kyphosis, sometimes referred to as a "dowager's hump."

Fractures in the upper thoracic spine may occur without a significant increase in discomfort, because of the support afforded by the rib cage; however, when crush fractures involve the lower thoracic or upper lumbar vertebrae, severe pain may result.

The patient, then, will present with the history of a grumbling debilitating back pain punctuated on occasion with one or more episodes of severe incapacitating pain. When the history is prolonged the patients may also relate progressive loss of height and rounding of the upper thoracic spine. On examination the thoracic kyphosis is noted with a compensatory increase in the lumbar lordosis. If, over a period of time, the patient has sustained several vertebral crush fractures, the rib cage may come to rest on the iliac crest.

X-rays of the spine show general loss of bone density and on closer inspection reveal lack of the horizontally disposed trabeculae. There may be ballooning of the discs into the vertebrae resulting in a fishtail appearance of the vertebral bodies. Compression fractures and end plate fractures are common.

Secondary osteoporosis may produce an identical radiological appearance, and it is important to exclude the possibility of systemic disease before making the diagnosis of primary osteoporosis.

Idiopathic osteoporosis does not produce any changes in the blood chemistry. Osteomalacia and hyperparathyroidism specifically affect calcium and phosphorous metabolism. Bone activity is reflected by the elevated alkaline phosphatase in both these conditions. Multiple myeloma, which may present with back pain and with an x-ray showing diffuse osteoporosis of the spine, is associated with significant changes in blood chemistry. There are alterations in the albumen and globulin ratios and abnormal globulins can be detected. The sedimentation rate is raised and frequently there is a significant anemia. The changes in the blood chemistry of these various conditions are summarized in table 3.2.

The treatment of postmenopausal or senile osteoporosis is frustratingly difficult. There is no evidence that any chemical therapy available to date or any replacement therapy reverses the metabolic change. The

Table 3.2. Hematological and Biochemical Changes in Common Types of Osteoporosis

	Osteoporosis	Osteomalacia	Hyperparathyroidism	Multiple Myeloma	Advanced Metastatic Disease
Hemogram				<10 gm%	↓
ESR*	No			↑↑↑	↑
BUN/CR	Abnormal			N↑	N↑
Calcium	Values	↓	↑	N↑	↑
Phosphorus		↓	N↓	↑	↓
Alkaline phosphatases		↑	↑	↑	↑
Acid phosphatases					↑ (prostate)
Uric acid			N↑	↑	↑
Protein electrophoresis				M spike	globulin
Immunoelectrophoresis				M spike	N/ABN

* ESR, erythrocyte sedimentation rate.

risks of many therapeutic measures advocated frequently outweigh any possible advantage. Estrogens have been given for the treatment of this condition. They are associated with the nuisance of withdrawal bleeding and the significant risk of deep vein thrombosis. Estrogen therapy does not reverse the calcium imbalance. Androgens and anabolic steroids are more likely to increase muscle bulk than bone bulk. The administration of fluorides is sometimes associated with some subjective improvement and an apparent, albeit slight, increase in bone density on x-ray.

This may be an artifact occasioned by the fact that fluoride salts are more radio-opaque.

It would seem logical to make more calcium available to the body, achieved by instructing the patients to drink 1 qt of skim milk and take 1 gm of calcium gluconate a day with 50,000 units of vitamin D once a week.

However, the body will not utilize this extra source of calcium unless a demand is created. This demand can only be created by increasing the patient's activities. This is the crux of treatment. Increased activity by increasing the functional capacity of the paraspinal muscles helps to decrease the venous congestion in the vertebral bodies and thereby helps to overcome the tiresome, constant, nagging discomfort these unfortunate souls experience. The increased demand on the bony skeleton resulting from increased physical activity helps to slow down the rate of bone resorption. The problem lies in devising methods to increase physical activity without subjecting the patients to an intolerable increase in discomfort.

In order to enable the patients to start on a program of increasing activities, it is necessary to give them sufficient analgesics to control the anticipated increase in pain. As in any chronic pain syndrome, the analgesics should be given on a time-dependent basis and not on demand. Ideally the analgesic should be given in a syrup form so that the physician has full control of the dosage. He can gradually reduce the amount of analgesic in each milliliter without the patient's knowledge and therefore without creating any apprehension.

Protected to some extent by the cover of analgesics, the patients can be started on a course of increasing activities. In many instances, it is necessary to enlist the aid of a physical therapist. Patients in whom pain is intensified by minimal activities may need the help of a therapeutic pool initially before starting on a graduated general exercise program. It is important to emphasize that these are general exercises, that is to say, exercises designed to build up muscle tone in all limbs, as well as building up the tone of the parasinal and abdominal muscles. Under instruction from the physical therapist and under the guidance of a physician, the patient should then start to increase daily activities around the home.

Some will need the assistance of a spinal support. If the patient is plump and the major pain is in the low back, a simple canvas corset reinforced with steel is all that is required. If the patient is very thin, such a garment will not give any support; therefore these patients will require a rigid thoracopelvic brace that grasps the pelvis and the lower thoracic cage firmly. Midthoracic pain aggravated by the tendency of the spine to droop forwards on prolonged activity requires a more rigid support. A Taylor brace is frequently prescribed. This brace leaves much to be desired. The rigid paraspinal vertical supports can be contoured to the spine, but the patient has to be held to these supports by straps that pass over the shoulders and under the axillae. They are, in effect, hung to a post. To give sufficient support, the straps should be tight and as such they constitute a tiresome yoke.

The patients are more comfortable if they are provided with a rigid thoracopelvic brace with a thoracic extension that the supports the sternum (fig. 3.9).

In a few the support afforded by braces of this type is not sufficient. They need to be held more firmly and consideration should be given to a form-fitting plastic brace. Before ordering such an expensive support, it is wise to ensure that it will give the desired relief. This is best decided by applying a well moulded plaster jacket. The patient can wear this for several days. If she finds that the support enables her to get around in greater comfort, then the plaster jacket can be used as a mould for the manufacture of a plastic body jacket. The physician should not regard the provision of a jacket, a brace, or a plastic body jacket as the end of treatment. The sole function of such supports is to enable the patient to become more active without increasing discomfort. The main direction of treatment remains the same: increase in general muscle tone, increase in

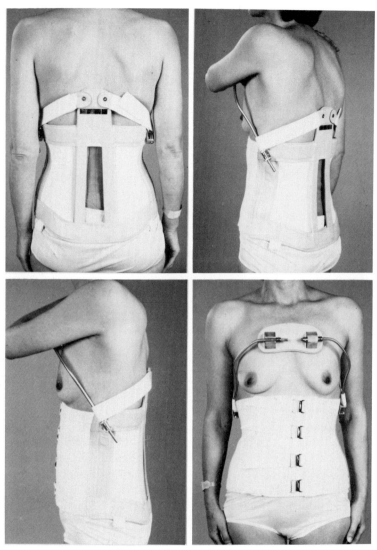

Fig. 3.9. Thoracopelvic brace.

strength of the paraspinal muscle, and increase in the activities of daily living.

These patients are frequently weary and near defeat. They need constant encouragement and frequent reassurance over a long period of time. The physician must ensure that such encouragement is given to them not only by himself, but also by the physical therapist and probably most important by all the members of the family.

CHAPTER 4

Spondylolisthesis

"False facts are highly injurious to progress of science, for they often endure long; but false views, if supported by some evidence do little harm, for everyone takes a salutary pleasure in proving their falseness."

—Charles Darwin

Scoliosis, spondylolysis, and spondylolisthesis are the major structural changes in the spine that may on occasion give rise to low back pain.

Scoliosis is a topic in itself and, therefore, is mentioned only when discussing the differential diagnosis of low back pain. Spondylolisthesis is more directly related to the low back pain syndrome and, therefore, merits more detailed description.

Herbineaux, a Belgian obstetrician, noted in 1782 that occasionally a bony prominence in front of the sacrum constituted an obstruction to labor. It has always been assumed that the condition he was describing was a complete spondylolisthesis, a spondyloptosis. He may be regarded as the first person to describe the lesion. Killian, who coined the term spondylolisthesis, felt that the lesion was due to a slow subluxation of the posterior facets. However, Robert theorized that the slip could not occur without a defect in the neural arch and the lesion was demonstrated 30 years later by Lambl. Neugebauer recognized the fact that the slip could occur with or without a defect in the neural arch. His work, unfortunately, was largely forgotten and subsequent interest became focused on the neural arch defect. The discussions on the nature, the etiology, the age of onset, and the radiological appearance of the defect obscured the fact that spondylolisthesis can, and does, occur with an intact neural arch. The management of painful spondylolisthesis obviously must depend on the type of lesion present; therefore, before discussing treatment, it is necessary to describe in detail the various types of spondylolisthesis.

Forward slip of the fifth vertebra is resisted by the bony block of the posterior facets, by the intact neural arch and pedicle, by normal bone plasticity preventing stretch of the pedicle, and by the intervertebral

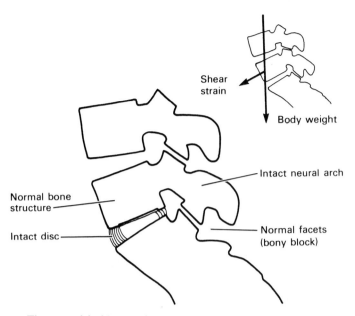

Shear strain

Body weight

Intact neural arch

Normal bone structure

Intact disc

Normal facets (bony block)

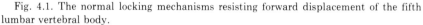

Fig. 4.1. The normal locking mechanisms resisting forward displacement of the fifth lumbar vertebral body.

discs bonding the vertebral bodies together (fig. 4.1). Breakdown of this normal locking mechanism occurs with articular defects and with defects in the neural arch. These pathological defects produce six recognizable clinical groups of spondylolisthesis: congenital, isthmic, spondylolytic, traumatic, degenerative, and pathological.

Congenital Spondylolisthesis

Congenital spondylolisthesis with forward displacement of a vertebral body being present at birth is a clinical curiosity. The spinal defect is usually only one of multiple congenital anomalies and the clinical problem presented is not the management of the spondylolisthesis, but the management of the associated congenital scoliosis.

Isthmic Spondylolisthesis

The basic lesion in isthmic spondylolisthesis appears to be an attenuation of the pars interarticularis which gets pulled out and thinned as though it were made of a malleable plastic. As the slip increases, and as the pars interarticularis becomes increasingly stretched, it may eventually break, but this break is secondary to the slip and is not the cause of the slip (fig. 4.2). On occasion, there may be a subluxation of the posterior joints between L5 and the sacrum due to a lack of development

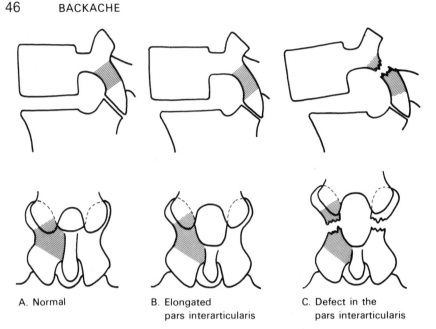

A. Normal   B. Elongated   C. Defect in the
pars interarticularis   pars interarticularis

Fig. 4.2. Isthmic spondylolisthesis. The pars interarticularis which was normal at birth (A) becomes attenuated and elongated allowing the vertebral body to slip forwards in relationship to the vertebral body below (B). Eventually on some occasions, the elongated pars interarticularis may break (C). This defect in the pars interarticularis is, however, secondary to the slip and is not the cause of the forward displacement of the vertebral body.

of the first sacral arch, with absence or dysplasia of the superior articular facets of the sacrum. The only structure preventing forward slip of the fifth lumbar vertebra is the lumbosacral disc. When this breaks down, the fifth lumbar vertebra slips forward with the inferior facets gliding over the rudimentary superior articular facets. The spinous process of L5 eventually comes to rest in the fibrous defect in the first sacral arch (fig. 4.3). However, this by itself would not allow a very marked slip. Further slipping must involve attenuation and elongation of the pars interarticularis.

In this form of spondylolisthesis, slipping occurs early in life and is permitted by virtue of detachment of the hyaline cartilage plate. The degree of slip is usually quite marked. In severe degrees of slip, the basic pathology is frequently overlooked because when severe degrees of slip are noted on x-ray it has always been assumed that there must be a defect in the pars interarticularis. The fact that the defect is not shown on the x-ray has been ascribed to difficulties in radiological techniques. The important clinical feature of the lesion is the lack of a defect in the pars interarticularis. Because there is no defect, the neural arch comes forward with the slipping vertebra and the cauda equina may be compressed between the laminae of L4 and L5 and the dorsal area of the first sacral body. Lane in 1893 described a young woman who had the misfortune to be the serving maid of a man who suffered from the delusion that life was all cricket. He would frequently strike her in the rear with a cricket bat which he always carried around with him. She gradually became paraplegic. Lane, describing his operative findings, stated that the neural arch was intact and as it had slipped forward had compressed the dura mater of the cauda equina. According to Lane, the spinous process of L5 lay in the fibrous defect of the dorsum of the sacrum. This is a beautiful description of the pathology of isthmic spondylolisthesis. Although examples of cauda equina compression are sometimes seen with this type of spondylolisthesis, the attenuation and elongation of the isthmus that inevitably occur usually prevent any significant distortion of the cauda equina (fig. 4.4). In fact, the majority of patients present without any evidence of nerve root irritation at all.

The average age for onset of symptoms is 14 in girls and 16 in boys. The onset may be quite sudden and dramatic and is aptly termed a "listhetic crisis." The patient experiences a sudden onset of backache and, on

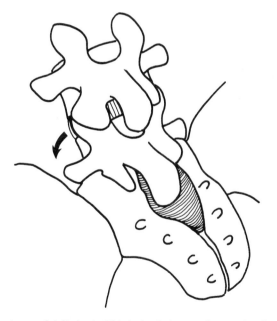

Fig. 4.3. Isthmic spondylolisthesis. This lesion is frequently associated with rudimentary superior articular facets of the sacrum. With degeneration of the lumbosacral disc, the fifth lumbar vertebra is displaced forwards in relation to the sacrum.

The spinous process of L5 eventually comes to rest in a fibrous defect usually present on the dorsal aspect of the first sacral arch.

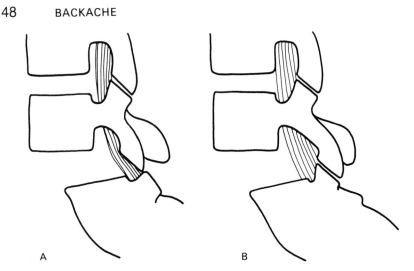

Fig. 4.4. Isthmic spondylolisthesis. In the presence of a normal pars interarticularis, forward dislocation of the fifth lumbar vertebra in relation to the sacrum is likely to produce compression of the cauda equina (A).

The elongation of the pars interarticularis associated with the forward displacement of the fifth lumbar vertebra in isthmic spondylolisthesis maintains the diameter of the spinal canal and obviates compression of the cauda equina (B).

examination, characteristically presents with a rigid lumbar spine which is commonly associated with a spastic or functional scoliosis. The pelvis is rotated anteriorly, giving rise to a flat sacrum; hamstring spasm is frequently seen, making the patient walk with bent knees (fig. 4.5).

The reason for differentiating this group of spondylolisthesis from the others is that the indications for surgery are much more clear-cut than in the next group, spondylolytic spondylolisthesis. If an isthmic spondylolisthesis goes to the stage of producing severe symptoms before the age of 21, with or without signs of nerve root irritation, it is unlikely that the patient will make a complete recovery without surgical intervention. Patients presenting with a first or even second degree slip will probably continue to slip more if seen in their early teens. There is evidence to substantiate the view that fusion performed at this stage will prevent further slip.

In the surgical management of this condition, the following points must be borne in mind. It is unwise to attempt to reduce the slip. Even if the slip is successfully reduced, it is most unlikely that the reduction will be held and, even so, nothing much has been achieved. Patients who present evidence of root tension or impairment of root conduction will require laminectomy and, on occasion, decompression of the involved root or roots. All will require stabilization and the best method of fusion devised to date is the ala transverse fusion (fig. 4.6).

Spondylolytic Spondylolisthesis

In spondylolytic spondylolisthesis, the basic lesion is a defect in the neural arch across the pars interarticularis (fig. 4.7). The etiology of this lesion is unknown. The neural arch defects occur most commonly between the ages of 5 and 7. Forward slipping of the vertebral body occurs most frequently between the ages of 10 and 15 and rarely increases after 20.

Despite the uncertainty as to the etiology of the neural arch defect, the radiological appearance is well known, perhaps too well known. The patient presenting with low back pain constitutes an irksome problem to the orthopedic surgeon. The diagnosis is usually obscure or cannot be proven. Treatment perforce is empirical, and the results of treatment, in many instances, are unrewarding. The demonstration, therefore, on x-ray of a gross abnormality of this type is generally greeted with a sigh of relief. Here is a recognizable cause of backache; here is an easily understood and treated lesion. However, a word of caution must be inter-

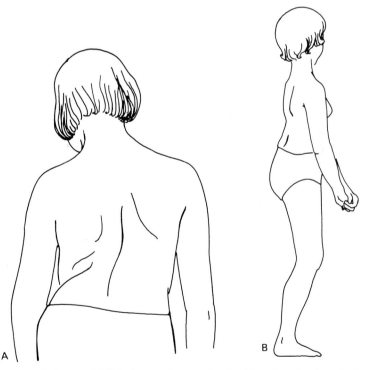

Fig. 4.5. A "listhetic crisis" is frequently associated with a functional scoliosis (A). Hamstring spasm is common despite anterior rotation of the pelvis, and the patient frequently stands and walks with bent knees (B).

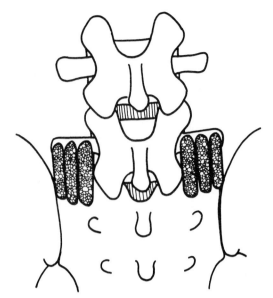

Fig. 4.6. Ala transverse fusion using corticocancellous grafts bridging the gap between the transverse process of L5 and the ala of the sacrum.

jected. Severe degrees of slip may be present in patients who engage in very vigorous activities and yet never suffer from backache.

Because there is no doubt that spondylolytic spondylolisthesis can, and does, occur without producing symptoms, the mere radiological demonstration of the defect in a patient with back pain does not indicate that the source of the symptoms has necessarily been demonstrated. Other anatomical variants have in the past been indicted as a cause of backache. It is now generally accepted that none of these anatomical variants is, by itself, a cause of low back pain. The question must arise, therefore, as to whether a neural arch defect, with or without a slip of the vertebral body, is yet another example of an anatomical variant incorrectly blamed as a cause of low back pain.

In examining this question further, it is important to take the following points into consideration. Stewart has shown that in some Eskimo communities the incidence of neural arch defects may rise as high as 50%. It is most unlikely that 50% of the Eskimos in these communities are severely handicapped by low back pain. The incidence of spondylolysis in the white population of the North American continent is about 6%. If neural arch defects were a common cause of low back pain, then the incidence of such defects in the backache population should be very much higher than 6%. However, an analysis of 996 adult patients with low back pain seen over the course of 1 year revealed an incidence of only

7.6%. This incidence is not significantly greater than the population as a whole. The analysis as it stands raises doubts as to whether neural arch defects are ever a source of symptoms. However, it is not unusual that patients with spondylolisthesis may become completely symptom-free following a successful spinal fusion. In trying to explain this apparent contradiction, patients with back pain were divided into three age groups (under 26, 26 to 39, and over 40) and the incidence of spondylolisthesis studied in each group (table 4.1). Over 40, the incidence was about the same as the population as a whole, whereas under 26, nearly 19%, a significant number, showed the defect. From this it can be said that if the x-ray of a patient with back pain shows a spondylolisthesis, then if the patient is under 26 the defect is probably the cause of the symptoms; between 26 and 40, it is only possibly the cause; over 40 it is rarely, if

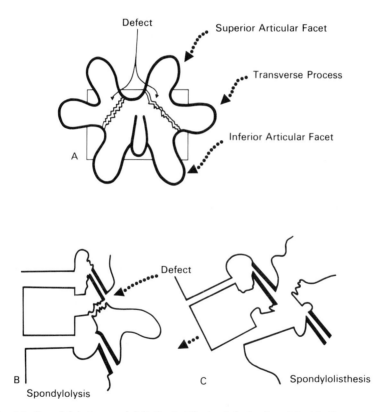

Fig. 4.7. Spondylolytic spondylolisthesis. The basic lesion is a defect in the neural arch across the pars interarticularis (A and B). When degenerative changes occur in the subjacent disc, the vertebral body will displace forwards carrying with it the superimposed spinal column and leaving behind the inferior articular facets, the lamina, and the spinous process (C).

ever, the sole cause of symptoms. In the management of spondylolisthesis associated with neural arch defects, the age of the patient, therefore, is of prime importance.

When considering the pathogenesis of symptoms in this group, the following points must be remembered. The lesion may be asymptomatic. If the syndesmosis firmly bonds the two halves of the neural arch together, there is no mechanical instability and probably no mechanical reason for pain. If, however, the syndesmosis is loose, separation occurs on flexion (fig. 4.8), and a strain is applied to the fibrous syndesmosis and to the supraspinous ligament as well. Repetitive strains of this nature could give rise both to local pain and referred pain in sciatic distribution.

Root irritation is not uncommon. With forward slip of the vertebral body, the intervertebral foramen is generally enlarged and the nerve root is not encroached upon because the neural arch is left behind as the vertebral body slips forward. However, nerve root compression can occur in the following circumstances. On occasion, when the vertebral body slips forward, the neural arch will rotate on the pivot formed by its

Table 4.1. Incidence of Spondylolisthesis

Age	No. of Patients	Arch Defects	Percentage
Under 25	116	22	18.9
26–39	350	26	7.6
Over 40	530	28	5.2
Total	996	76	7.6

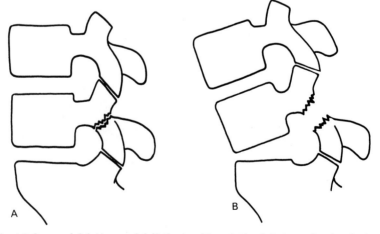

Fig. 4.8. In spondylolytic spondylolisthesis, although the defect may be closed when the patient holds the spine in extension (A), separation may occur to a marked degree on flexion (B).

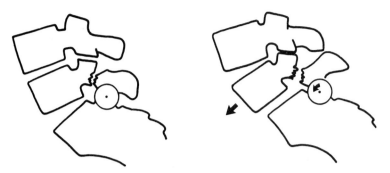

Fig. 4.9. When the vertebral body slips forward, the traction applied to the free neural arch may cause it to rotate on the pivot formed by its articulation with the sacrum. When this occurs the anterior aspect of the neural arch defect may encroach upon the foramen and compress the emerging nerve root.

articulation with the sacrum and may encroach upon the foramen (fig. 4.9). Small ossicles are frequently found on the anterior aspect of the isthmic defect and, when these are present, there is greater likelihood of root compression by the rotated free neural arch. The likelihood of foraminal entrapment of the nerve root is increased if a traction spur develops on the posterior border of the vertebral body after it has slipped forward. The superior portion of the pars interarticularis may also encroach on the foramen.

The nerve root, after it has emerged through the intervertebral foramen, is more or less fixed as it courses through the large muscle masses. With spondylolisthesis the vertebral body glides forward and downward along the inclined plane of the superior surface of the vertebral body below. This downward drop is particularly marked at L5-S1. With this movement of the vertebra, the pedicles descend on the nerve roots and kink them as they emerge through the foramen (fig. 4.10).

Forward slipping will not occur without degenerative changes occurring in the underlying disc. This generally takes place as a slow attrition of the disc, but sometimes the disc collapses and bulges out around the periphery of the vertebral body just like squashed putty. The nerve root may get buried in this bulging mass after it has emerged from the foramen.

There is a strong ligamentous band that runs from the undersurface of the transverse process to the side of the vertebral body, the corporotransverse ligament (fig. 4.11). At L5, the fifth lumbar nerve root runs between the ligament and the ala of the sacrum. With marked forward slip and downward descent of L5, the ligament comes down like a guillotine on the fifth lumbar root and may entrap it against the ala of the sacrum.

Kinking of the nerve root by the pedicle and extraforaminal entrap-

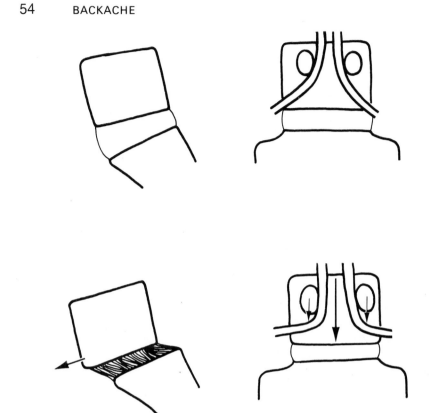

Fig. 4.10. Kinking of the nerve roots by the pedicles as the body of L5 slips downward and forward.

ment of the nerve all involve the nerve emerging through the foramen at the site of the slip. With slipping of the fifth lumbar vertebra, it is the fifth lumbar root that is involved. A possible cause of fifth lumbar root compression in patient with an L5-S1 slip is, of course, a disc herniation at L4-L5. However, in a patient with an L5-S1 slip presenting L5 root signs, if the myelogram does not reveal any defect, then pedicular kinking or extraforaminal compression must be considered as the possible source of the clinical signs.

Spondylolysis predisposes to premature disc degeneration in the subjacent disc and spondylolisthesis does not occur without disc degeneration. These degenerative changes may of themselves be painful, giving rise to local or referred pain in sciatic distribution without root irritation.

The local causes of pain then in spondylolysis, with or without a slip, are instability, foraminal encroachment of the nerve root, extraforaminal entrapment of the nerve root, and disc degeneration.

Over the age of 30, other sources of pain become increasingly common and these must perforce influence treatment. A disc rupture may occur in association with spondylolisthesis. Although it may occur at the segment below the slip, much more commonly it is seen at the disc above the slip. When a disc rupture occurs at the segment above the slipping vertebra, one has to accept the fact that the patient's symptoms may be stemming solely from the herniated disc and that the spondylolisthesis may be asymptomatic. In some instances, discectomy alone is sufficient

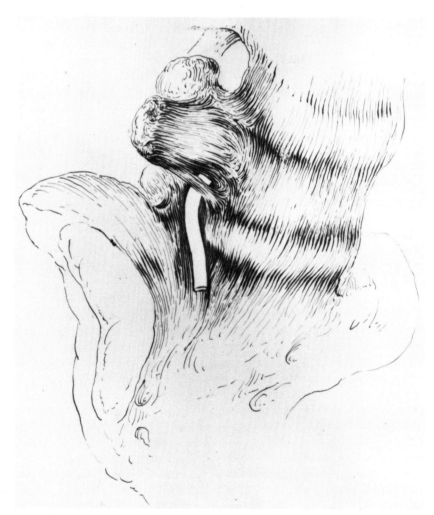

Fig. 4.11. The relationship of the fifth lumbar nerve root to the corporotransverse ligamment.

to give complete relief of symptoms. This is particularly true in patients who have never experienced any back disability previously.

Symptomatic disc degeneration, as distinct from disc herniation, may occur above the level of the slip. This may produce local pain, pain referred in sciatic distribution, or referred pain only.

Unlike isthmic spondylolisthesis in which severe slips are associated with pelvic rotation and flattening of the back, in spondylolytic spondylolisthesis a forward slip of more than 50% is frequently associated with hyperlordosis. When this occurs, the hyperlordosis, by itself, may cause part or all of the symptoms complained of and the symptoms derived from this source will, of course, persist after a spinal fusion.

With long-standing lumbosacral pathology, the lumbodorsal junction becomes the site of maximal movement, and in patients over 35, degenerative changes of a marked degree are frequently seen in the discs and posterior joints in this area. Degenerative changes in this region may present with low back pain as the sole symptom. The fact that changes at the lumbodorsal junction play a role in the production of the patient's low back pain can be demonstrated on clinical examination. With the patient lying on his side with hips and knees flexed to flatten the lumbar curve, the examiner applies firm lateral pressure to the spinous processes of the vertebrae at the lumbodorsal junction. If there is disc instability at this region, then when pressure is applied to the spinous processes and maintained for a moment, the patient will experience pain referred down to the lumbosacral region.

It must always be remembered that a spondylolisthesis may be asymptomatic; consequently, the possibility of other sources of back pain must never be forgotten.

In summary, when a patient with low back pain demonstrates a spondylolisthesis on x-ray, the following points must be borne in mind. The spondylolisthesis may be asymptomatic and the back pain may stem from causes outside the spine.

If the pain is indeed spinal in origin, it may be due to instability at the defect, root pressure due to disc herniation above or below the slip, foraminal encroachment of the nerve root, or extraforaminal entrapment of the nerve root. The pain, however, may arise elsewhere in the spine, being due to disc degeneration above the slip, hyperlordosis, or thoraco-lumbar disc degeneration. Finally, the pain may stem from an entirely unrelated cause, such as a secondary deposit in the spine.

Even if the patient's symptoms are indeed due to the spinal lesion, the mere radiological demonstration of a spondylolysis or spondylolisthesis does not indicate that operative intervention is mandatory. There are, of course, certain unusual instances in which operative intervention is unavoidable, such as evidence of cauda equina compression, or evidence of unresolving or increasing impairment of root conduction. Apart from such examples, primary treatment should be conservative. Unlike isthmic spondylolisthesis, further slipping is unlikely to occur, and surgery, therefore, is not indicated to prevent further forward displacement. Continuing disabling pain constitutes the sole indication for surgery in this group of patients.

The type of surgical intervention required demands very careful evaluation of the patient. If the patient presents evidence of root tension or impairment of root conduction, the level of the lesion must be determined by clinical examination and confirmed by myelography. In instances of foraminal encroachment of the root, diagnostic root sleeve infiltration is a very useful ancillary measure. The technique of nerve root infiltration is described in chapter 10. When the patient's complaints are mainly of pain of sciatic distribution due to foraminal encroachment of the fifth lumbar root, a foraminotomy may be all that is required. The decision to fuse the spine is determined by a history of repeated episodes or continuing back pain of incapacitating severity.

Discography is of inestimable value in determining the extent of fusion required. If the discs above the level of an L5-S1 slip are normal on discography, a localized lumbosacral fusion is all that is required. The most reliable method of obtaining a single segment fusion in slips up to 50% is to fuse the transverse process of L5 to the ala of the sacrum. In males over 18 a pedicled bone graft can be swung from the posterior superior iliac crest to the transverse process (fig. 4.12). This type of spinal fusion, however, should never be performed in females in the child-bearing age because the sacroiliac joints are fused by this technique.

When the forward displacement is more than half the width of the sacrum or when discography reveals degenerative changes at the L4-L5 disc, the fusion must be extended up to the transverse process of L4.

The necessity for a three-segment fusion arises from time to time, for example, a spondylolysis of the last three lumbar segments. A similar problem is presented by an L5-S1 slip with symptomatic degenerative changes at L3-L4 and L4-L5, and L4-L5 slip with disc degenerative changes at the segments above and below the slip, or an L3-L4 lesion with symptomatic degenerative changes in the subjacent discs (fig. 4.13). Reviews of three-segment fusions for disc degeneration reveal a pseudarthrosis rate of 40%. To avoid this high pseudarthrosis rate, these cases should be treated by a circumferential fusion. A posterior and intertransverse fusion is first performed and 3 weeks later, an anterior interbody fusion is performed at the L3-L4 and L4-L5 levels. An anterior fusion at the L5-S1 segment is not required because in triple segment fusions when a pseudarthrosis develops, it is always seen at the upper levels. This is a

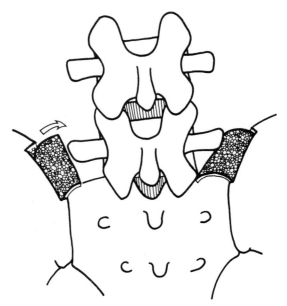

Fig. 4.12. Iliotransverse fusion. A flap of bone attached at its base is swung down from the inner table of the iliac crest and is placed in firm contact with the transverse process of L5 and the ala of the sacrum.

formidable procedure and the patient must be completely incapacitated by his symptoms to justify the operation.

Traumatic Spondylolisthesis

Forward slipping of a vertebral body may occur as the result of a dislocation of the posterior joints, or because of a fracture of a spinous process extending into the lamina at the pars interarticularis. These are really examples of fracture dislocations of the spine and should not be classified as traumatic spondylolisthesis. A fracture through the pars interarticularis with forward slip of the vertebral body, a true traumatic spondylolisthesis, is rare. When a patient who has been involved in a severe accident demonstrates a spondylolisthesis on x-ray, it is difficult to say whether this is a patient with a pre-existing spondylolisthesis who has been involved in an accident. Clearly defined edges of the vertebral body of L5 and a sharply pointed anterior margin of the sacrum are both suggestive of an acute lesion. In contradistinction to spondylolytic and isthmic spondylolisthesis, an acute traumatic slip can be reduced and can be maintained in the reduced position.

A neural arch defect across the pars interarticularis may also occur on rare occasions as a result of trauma, either from a forced hyperextension or from a forced flexion strain. Here again, the problem always arises as to whether the defect resulted from the accident or whether the patient had the defect prior to the accident. The sites and types of defects are frequently unusual. Healing of the lesion on immobilization is irrefutable evidence of the traumatic origin of the lesion.

Degenerative Spondylolisthesis

Junghanns, in 1929, reported 14 instances of spondylolisthesis found in autopsy specimens without any defect in the neural arch. He coined the

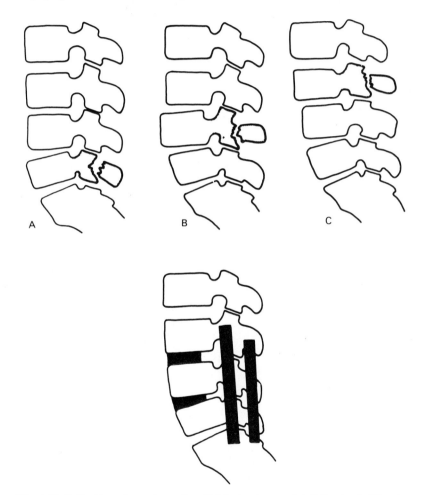

Fig. 4.13. Indications for a circumferential fusion in spondylolisthesis. *A*, Disc degeneration at two segments above slip; *B*, disc degeneration at segment above and below slip; and, *C*, disc degeration at the two segments below slip.

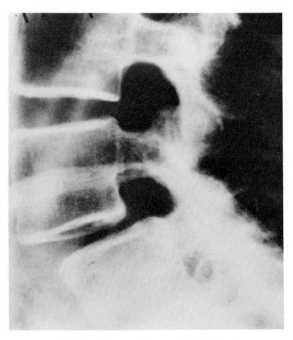

Fig. 4.14. Degenerative spondylolisthesis.

term pseudospondylolisthesis. The slip is never very great (fig. 4.14). It most commonly occurs at L4. The L4-L5 segment of the lumbar spine is normally the site of the greatest mobility, and in L4-L5 degenerative spondylolisthesis it is frequently associated with excessive mobility or even with a backward and forward piston-like movement on flexion and extension (fig. 4.15). It is probably this excessive movement that causes the breakdown in the posterior joints in these slips. Females predominate with the average age of onset of symptoms about 50. This form of spondylolisthesis is really a manifestation of disc degeneration which may produce back pain because of the gross segmental instability and associated posterior joint damage. On occasion, root entrapment may be produced by a combination of a diffuse annular bulge at the level of the slip, shingling of the laminae, and buckling of the ligamentum flavum. The spinal canal is further narrowed by subluxation of the posterior joints which are enlarged by osteophytic outgrowths. All these factors combine to produce entrapment of the nerve roots as they course through the subarticular gutter. This is a form of segmental spinal stenosis.

In summary, the nature of the lesion and the pathogenesis of the lesion make it obvious that the management of degenerative spondylolisthesis

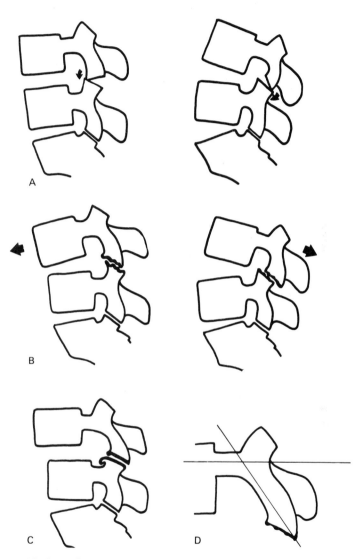

Fig. 4.15. Mechanical insufficiency of an intervertebral disc permits excessive movement on flexion and extension (A). The posterior joints undergo degenerative changes because of this abnormal movement and with increasing breakdown permit forward and backward gliding of the involved vertebral bodies (B).

Subluxation of the arthritic zygapophysial joints permits forward displacement of the vertebral body (C), and the displacement becomes fixed because of an increase in the angle between the pedicle and the inferior processes (D).

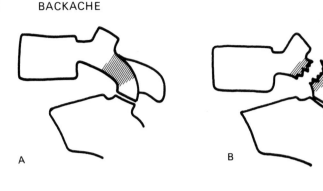

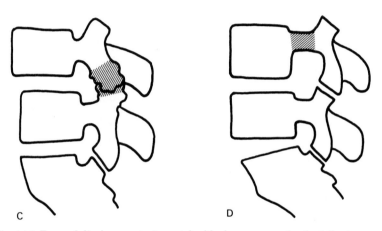

Fig. 4.16. Forward displacement of a vertebral body may occur for the following reasons: A, elongation of the pars interarticularis (isthmic spondylolisthesis); B, a bilateral neural arch defect (spondylolytic spondylolisthesis); C, subluxation of degenerated zygapophysial joints (degenerative spondylolisthesis); or D, elongation of the pedicles (pathological spondylolisthesis).

is indeed just the management of degenerative disc disease with or without nerve root irritation.

Pathological Spondylolisthesis

On occasion, generalized bone disease such as osteogenesis imperfecta, osteomalacia, achondroplasia, or a localized bony change such as a secondary deposit or Paget's disease may allow attenuation of the *pedicles* and thereby allow the vertebral body to slip forward. It is to be noted that, unlike the other types of spondylolisthesis, forward displacement of the vertebral body in pathological spondylolisthesis is permitted by elongation of the pedicle (fig. 4.16). Obviously the management of the local lesion in this group of cases depends on the management of the cause of the primary disease.

Summary

Although spondylolisthesis presents a dramatic picture on x-ray, it may be asymptomatic and remain asymptomatic for the lifetime of the patient.

When the lesion does indeed produce symptoms, the pathogenesis of the symptoms (instability, root compression, etc.) must be established before treatment is instituted.

CHAPTER 5

Lesions of the Sacroiliac Joints

"Who is this that darkeneth counsel by words without knowledge."

—Job 38:2

Affections of the sacroiliac joints can be discussed under the headings of sprains, instability, inflammation, and infections.

SACROILIAC SPRAINS

The concept of a "sacroiliac sprain" as a common cause of backache and sciatica was introduced by Goldthwaite and Osgood in 1905. The common findings in patients suffering from mechanical backache, of pain situated over the sacroiliac joint and tenderness in this region, have tended to perpetuate this concept. However, this finding is usually a manifestation of the confusing phenomenon of referred pain. Mechanical lesions of the lumbosacral junction associated with disc degeneration frequently give rise to pain referred to the sacroiliac region and such patients will exhibit local tenderness here. It is understandably tempting to ascribe these findings to a pathological lesion in the underlying sacroiliac joint. However, the true source of this type of pain can be demonstrated by its experimental reproduction on injection of the supraspinous ligaments at the lumbosacral junction with hypertonic saline and by reproduction of the pain on discography of the L4-L5 and L5-S1 discs.

The anatomical configuration of the components of the sacroiliac joint makes the joint extremely stable (see fig. 1.13), and this inherent stability is reinforced by the powerful, massive posterior interosseus ligaments and by the strong accessory ligaments, the iliolumbar, the sacrotuberous, and the sacrospinous ligaments.

Over the age of 45—the backache years—in 30% of the population, the anterior capsule of the sacroiliac joint is ossified and, in these patients at least, the sacroiliac joints may be exonerated from the blame of backache. Under this age, minimal sliding and rotary movements occur, but considerable force, such as generated by falls from heights or motor vehicle injuries, is required to push the sacroiliac joints beyond their physiologically permitted range.

Violence of this degree will usually be associated with a fracture of the pelvis, but, in the unusual circumstances in which the whole brunt of the blow is absorbed by the supporting ligamentous structures of the sacroiliac joint, the findings are specific and pathognomonic:

1. There is tenderness over the lower third of the sacroiliac joint below the posterior inferior iliac spine.

2. The pubic symphysis is tender on palpation. The pelvis is a closed ring and cannot undergo stretching at one site only. In the absence of a fracture of the pelvic ring, if the sacroiliac joint is displaced the pubic symphysis must also suffer some disruption (fig. 5.1).

3. The clinically experienced symptoms may be reproduced on stressing the sacroiliac joint by any of the following maneuvers:

    a. Lateral manual compression of the iliac crest (fig. 5.2).

    b. Resisted abduction of the hip joint. When the gluteus medius contracts to abduct the hip, it pulls the ilium away from the sacrum. With sacroiliac joint lesions, abduction against resistance is painful (fig. 5.3).

    c. Hyperextension of the hip on the affected side against a stabilized pelvis. Although this maneuver, Gaenslen's test, was originally described for eliciting sacroiliac joint pain, the test is not specific. Hyperextension of the hip performed in this manner will also be painful in the presence of pre-existing hip disease, and patients suffering from irritation of the fourth lumbar nerve root

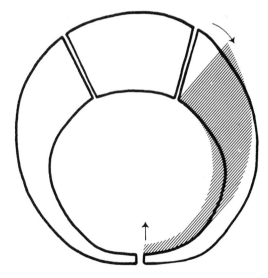

Fig. 5.1. Diagram showing that any movement of the sacroiliac joint must be associated with corresponding displacement at the symphysis pubis.

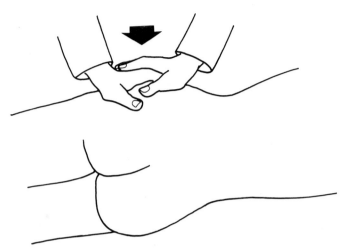

Fig. 5.2. With the patient lying on his side, the sacroiliac joint can be stressed by manually applying compression to the pelvis.

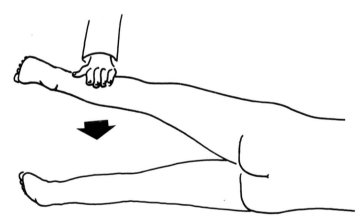

Fig. 5.3. In the absence of hip joint disease, pain experienced over the sacroiliac joint on resisted abduction of the leg is highly suggestive of a sacroiliac joint lesion.

may experience anterior thigh pain on this form of hyperextension of the hip (fig. 5.4).

4. Patients with painful sacroiliac joints may develop gluteal inhibition with a resulting Trendelenburg lurch on walking (fig. 5.5).

During the latter months of pregnancy, the supporting ligaments of the sacroiliac joints become "relaxed" to allow enlargement of the birth canal. At this point of time and during parturition, the joints are indeed susceptible to strain as a result of trivial trauma. The patients complain

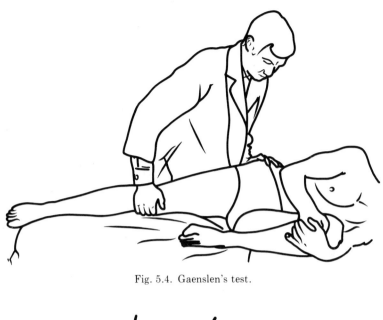

Fig. 5.4. Gaenslen's test.

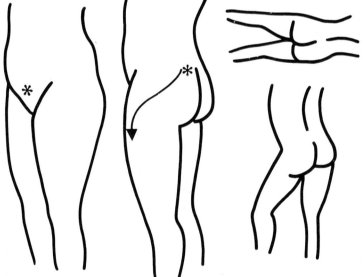

Fig. 5.5. Summary of findings in sacroiliac joint disease. Tenderness can be elicited not only over the sacroiliac joint, but over the symphysis pubis as well. The pain usually radiates over the lateral aspect of the great trochanter and down the front of the thigh. The patients exhibit pain on abduction of the hip on the affected side and walk with a Trendelenburg lurch.

of pain localized to the involved sacroiliac joint and the pain radiates around the greater trochanter and down the anterolateral aspect of the thigh. The patients present, on examination, the specific physical findings described above.

The symptoms of true sacroiliac sprains generally subside rapidly with bedrest, analgesics, and anti-inflammatory medications. The use of a trochanteric belt can give relief while walking and obviate the antalgic gait (fig. 5.6). In a few patients whose symptoms persist, intra-articular steroids may be necessary.

In summary then, it is worth repeating that sacroiliac strains, apart from those following parturition, are excessively rare, although commonly diagnosed. The concept of a sacroiliac strain is yet another example of how the phenomenon of referred pain and tenderness has clouded and confused the recognition of the pathological basis of spondylogenic pain. The sacroiliac region is a common site for referred pain and tenderness derived from segmental discogenic backache. The mere complaint of pain over the sacroiliac joint and the demonstration of local tenderness do not justify the diagnosis of a sacroiliac sprain.

The diagnosis is not justifiable unless the patient presents, in addition, pain on resisted abduction of the leg, pain on weight bearing on the affected extremity, tenderness over the symphysis pubis, and a Trendelenburg lurch. Additional evidence for the diagnosis can be gleaned by the temporary relief of discomfort afforded by wearing a very tight 2-inch

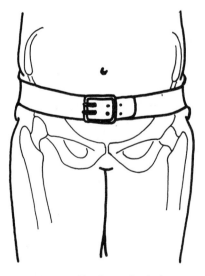

Fig. 5.6. Trochanteric cinch.

webbing belt placed around the pelvis between the iliac crest and the greater trochanter, the so-called "trochanteric cinch."

SACROILIAC INSTABILITY

Patients whose backache can be attributed to gross sacroiliac instability will give the history of preceding violent trauma resulting in disruption of the pelvic ring. The pain derived from this form of instability is disabling. It is refractory to conservative treatment and can only be treated by sacroiliac fusion.

A major stabilizer of the sacroiliac joint is the iliolumbar ligament. Destruction of this ligament during the course of removing a bone graft from the iliac crest may, on occasion, give rise to sacroiliac instability. The clinical picture may be confused because the patient will be complaining of pain over the donor site, but the characteristic radiation of pain down the anterolateral aspect of the thigh differentiates it from the all too common "donor site pain."

On examination, sacroiliac stress tests evoke a painful response. A palpable click over the symphysis pubis with alternate leg standing may be demonstrated. X-rays of the pelvis demonstrate the encroachment of the donor site into the sacroiliac joint. Occasionally, the symphysis pubis will show cyst formation and abnormal excursion when anteroposterior views of the pelvis are taken while the patient performs alternate leg standing.

INFLAMMATORY LESIONS OF THE SACROILIAC JOINT

Although present concepts of the etiology of back pain have deposed sacroiliac strains from their previous pre-eminence, nevertheless, in the assessment of patients with persisting back pain of obscure etiology, the clinician must always bear in mind the possibility of an inflammatory lesion of the sacroiliac joint, sacroiliitis. Sacroiliitis, presenting as back pain, is seen in ankylosing spondylitis, and it is also seen as a part of the skeletal manifestations of psoriasis and Reiter's syndrome.

Ankylosing Spondylitis

At one time ankylosing spondylitis was regarded as the spinal variant of rheumatoid arthritis. However, there are many factors that distinguish the two diseases. The sex incidence is different. Unlike rheumatoid arthritis, ankylosing spondylitis affects men in their second to third decade of life. The latex fixation test is rarely positive in ankylosing spondylitis.

Genetic factors appear to be of great importance because the disease is 20 times more common among relatives of patients with ankylosing spondylitis. In this regard there is one serological study that is of considerable interest. It has been determined that tissue rejection phenomena are dependent on genetically determined antigens on the surface of the leukocytes. One of these human leukocyte antigens (HLA W27) is present in 90% of patients with ankylosing spondylitis, whereas it is only found in 8% of the Caucasian population as a whole. African blacks do not suffer from ankylosing spondylitis and, interestingly enough, they do not have an HLA W27 antigen.

The lesion almost invariably starts in the sacroiliac joints and then extends upward to involve the spine at increasingly higher levels. In 5% the disease may originate in the thoracic spine and in about 13%, in the cervical spine. The costovertebral joints and the manubriosternal joint are involved early, and these changes account for the classical clinical sign of decreased chest expansion. The progress of the lesion and its major pathological features are well demonstrated on repeated x-ray examinations.

The first characteristic change may be best described as "fuzziness" of the sacroiliac joint (fig. 5.7). Oblique views of the sacroiliac joints initially show widening of the joint space produced by inflammatory destruction of the subarticular bone and subsequently progress through

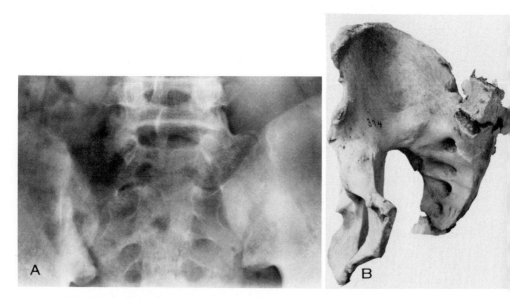

Fig. 5.7. *A*, X-ray demonstrating the irregular definition ("fuzziness") of the sacroiliac joints commonly seen in the early stages of ankylosing spondylitis.

B, In the later stages of the disease, the sacroiliac joint is completely obliterated by a bony ankylosis as shown in this specimen.

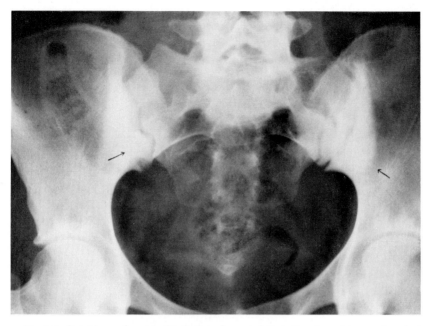

Fig. 5.8. Osteitis condensans ilii. It is to be noted that the area of bone sclerosis is confined to the iliac side of the sacroiliac joint.

the stages of subchondral sclerosis involving the iliac and sacral sides of the joint. This radiological change must be distinguished from osteitis condensans ilii. In this lesion, almost invariably found in multiparous women, there is a wedge-shaped area of sclerosis *confined to the iliac side of the joint* (fig. 5.8). It should be noted that there is no evidence that osteitis condensans ilii is ever a source of low back pain.

Radiological changes in the vertebral column are seen later in the disease process. There is "squaring" of the vertebral bodies most apparent on the lateral view (fig. 5.9). Later the outermost fibers of the annulus ossify, progressing eventually to complete ossification of the investing ligaments and giving rise to the so-called bamboo spine (fig. 5.10).

The disease is not confined to the musculoskeletal system. These unfortunate souls may have symptoms referable to their cardiovascular system (cardiac enlargement, conduction defects, pericarditis, and aortic insufficiency). One-quarter of the patients, on close questioning, will give a history of iritis and may, therefore, confuse the diagnosis with Reiter's syndrome. Ankylosing spondylitis may be associated with pulmonary fibrosis which combined with the marked decrease in rib cage movement may lead to significant loss of pulmonary function.

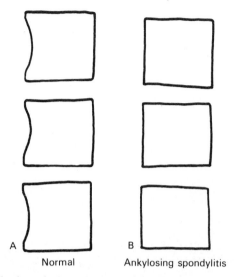

A   Normal

B   Ankylosing spondylitis

Fig. 5.9. A, The lateral view of a normal lumbar vertebral body presents a slight concavity anteriorly. B, In the early stages of ankylosing spondylitis, this concavity is filled in with the result that the vertebrae appear to be "squared off."

In the early stages of the process, the clinician is presented with a grumbling young man complaining of a grumbling stiff back. On examination it is noted that the lumbar spinous processes do not separate very well on forward flexion and the chest expansion is less than one would expect. Diminution of the chest expansion is a cardinal and important feature, and is the reason that assessment of chest expansion should always be part of the routine examination of a patient with backache.

The sedimentation rate may be slightly elevated, but all other routine laboratory investigations are within normal limits.

In attempting to establish the diagnosis in the early stages of the disease, x-ray assessment of the sacroiliac joints is of vital importance. It should be emphasized that by the time significant changes are noted in the vertebral column on x-ray the diagnosis of the condition should be very apparent on clinical examination alone. It is in the early stages, with changes confined to the sacroiliac joints, that a thorough radiological assessment is of great importance. The radiological abnormalities may be minimal and of questionable significance. Good quality x-rays must be obtained, supplemented, if necessary, by tomography. Further evidence of the nature of the lesion may, on occasion, be obtained from x-ray examination of the manubriosternal joint (fig. 5.11).

If the x-rays of the sacroiliac joints, the manubriosternal joints, and the lumbar spine appear to be within normal limits, but the symptoms persist, radiological examination should be repeated in 3 months. It is important to emphasize that the disease may be extremely slowly progressive and radiological changes correspondingly slow to develop. One of my patients was investigated in hospital annually over a period of 3 years. On each occasion, because it was felt that the disabling symptoms were discogenic in origin, diagnostic discography was undertaken. On each occasion the discograms were normal. Four years from the onset of symptoms of sufficient severity to prevent him from working, changes in the sacroiliac joints were noted on x-ray irrefutably indicative

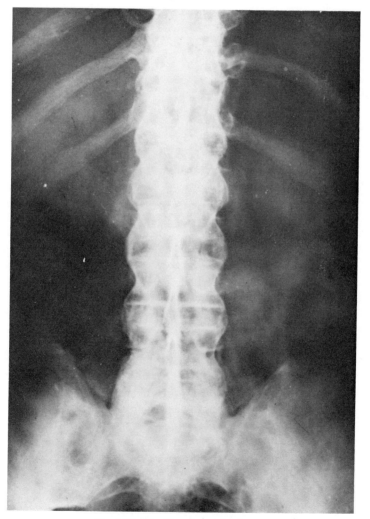

Fig. 5.10. The "bamboo spine."

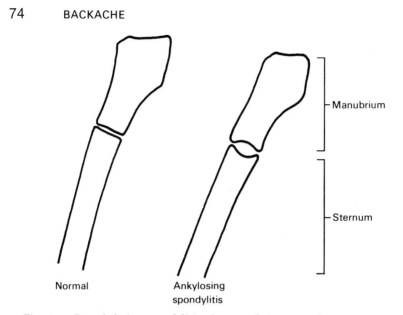

Fig. 5.11. In ankylosing spondylitis the manubriostructural joint may present a biconcave appearance on x-ray.

of ankylosing spondylitis! This is an extremely rare example. However, in the early stages of the disease, with minimal unrecognized or unrecognizable radiological changes, the patient does indeed stand in danger of being deposited in the diagnostic garbage can of incurable neuroses. Perhaps such patients may be protected in the future by the presence of the antigen HLA W27 which, although not diagnostic in itself, may well make the physician wary of the possibility of ankylosing spondylitis (fig. 5.12).

When considering treatment and in particular the advice that must be given to patients, it is important to have some knowledge of the natural history of the disease. The concept that the disease progresses to complete ankylosis with eventual relief of pain is not correct. The rapidity of development and the extent of involvement are totally unpredictable. Approximately 40% of patients undergo a benign course with an insidious onset of mild intermittent backache settling with time. In these patients the radiographic changes may be minimal and remain confined to the sacroiliac joints. Such patients can usually lead a reasonably normal life. Half of the patients have a severe clinical course with varying degrees of complete disease expression, and the remainder demonstrate a fulminating pattern to severe and permanent disability and a life of perpetual valetudinarianism.

The patient must be seen over a period of time before the clinician is able to give even a guarded prognosis.

No specific treatment of a curative nature presently exists. The role of the physician is diagnostic awareness of the disease, amelioration of the symptoms with the carefully controlled exhibition of anti-inflammatory medications, patient education, attention to the possibility of spinal deformities, and the management of peripheral joint arthropathies.

It is essential for the patient to understand the natural history of his disease in order that he understands the need for reasonable rest and a continuing program of postural education and exercises.

The exercise program is designed to maintain a straight spine or to attempt to increase lumbar lordosis. Every attempt must be made to maintain the already reduced respiratory excursion.

Occasionally, despite anti-inflammatory medication and despite excellent continued physical therapy, the spinal deformities progress relentlessly and inexorably to a stage at which the patient can only see a few feet in front of him when standing and may have difficulty in sitting and eating.

In such instances, surgical correction of the deformities must be considered. Operative correction is undertaken at the site of the maximal deformity, taking into full account the serious surgical hazards of

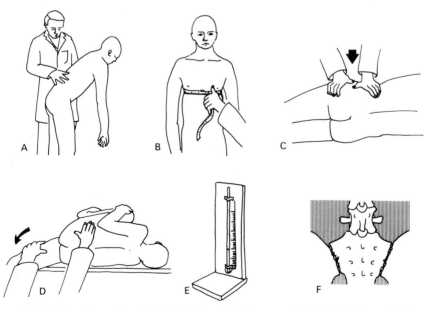

Fig. 5.12. Summary of major findings in ankylosing spondylitis. A, Rigidity of lumbar spine on forward flexion; B, decrease in chest expansion; C, pain on side-to-side compression of the pelvis; D, pain on Gaenslen's test; E, elevated sedimentation rate; and F, "fuzziness" of sacroiliac joints on x-ray.

respiratory problems and the danger of producing irreversible neurological damage (fig. 5.13).

Spondylitis Associated with Chronic Inflammatory Bowel Disease

It has been found that spondylitis and a peripheral seronegative arthritis occur in 5 to 20% of patients suffering from regional enteritis and chronic ulcerative colitis.

The etiology and pathogenesis of the peripheral arthropathy are unknown. Several distinguishing features have been noted: the acute onset, involvement of weight-bearing joints, a migratory pattern, and a short-lived course. The spondylitis is clinically and roentgenographically indistinguishable from idiopathic ankylosing spondylitis. In this regard,

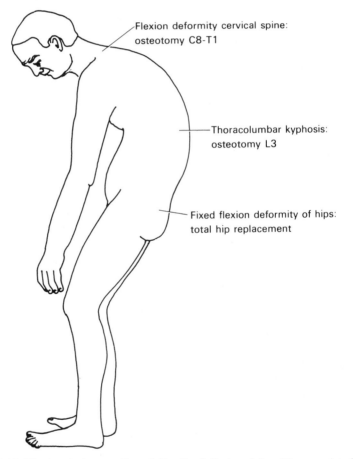

Fig. 5.13. The surgical correction of the fixed flexion deformities associated with ankylosing spondylitis is dependent on the type and site of the maximal deformity.

it is interesting to note that nearly 80% of the patients with spondylitis associated with inflammatory bowel disease are HLA W27-positive.

If a patient being treated for Crohn's disease or ulcerative colitis subsequently develops a grumbling backache, the possibility of sacroiliitis with spondylitis must be suspected. One must be aware that spondylitis can occur before the onset of intestinal disease and does so in at least one-third of the instances. Whereas the severity of the arthropathy correlates with the activity of the bowel disease, the spondylitis appears to progress independently of the primary lesion, and medical and surgical treatment of the bowel disease does not alter its progression.

Spondylitis Associated with Psoriasis

Almost identical radiological changes in the sacroiliac joints and lumbar spine may be seen in patients suffering from psoriatic arthritis. The age of onset of psoriatic arthritis is generally in the second or third decade, with women being more commonly afflicted than men. The etiology and pathogenesis have not been clarified. It is interesting to note that, on tissue typing, 60% of the patients with psoriatic arthritis, 90% of patients with psoriatic sacroiliac joint arthritis, and 100% of patients with psoriatic spondylitis present an HLA W27 antigen.

The clinician must always be mindful of the fact that the skin lesion of psoriasis does not protect patients from developing simple mechanical backache. Not every patient with psoriasis and back pain is suffering from spondylitis; nevertheless, if the patient has a peripheral arthritis, the possibility of a psoriatic sacroiliitis or spondylitis must be suspected and appropriate x-rays ordered.

Spondylitis Associated with Reiter's Syndrome

Back pain may be the presenting symptom of Reiter's syndrome. It is difficult to define Reiter's disease precisely. Classically it is the triad of nonbacterial urethritis, arthritis, and conjunctivitis. The onset is most common between the ages of 20 and 40, with males predominately affected. Episodes of extramarital sexual intercouse may precede attacks and the patients tend to be "sexual giants." The etiology of the disease is unknown, but evidence tends to indict an infectious agent.

Any one of the triad may be the presenting manifestation, although urethritis is by far the most common initial feature. The arthritis is marked by acute onset and by asymmetrical involvement of a few joints. The large weight-bearing joints, the joints of the midfoot, and the metatarsophalangeal and interphalangeal joints of the toes are the most commonly afflicted.

A high percentage of patients with Reiter's syndrome show radiographic evidence of sacroiliitis, but it is only a small percentage that develop a spondylitis. When spondylitis occurs, it is late in the disease evolution and is noted, therefore, as an association rather than a presenting finding.

INFECTIONS OF THE SACROILIAC JOINTS

In the past, tuberculosis was the most common cause of infective arthritis of the sacroiliac joints. Recently, an increasing frequency of pyogenic involvement has been noted, especially in children. The clinical picture is unfortunately vague. There is pain and tenderness over the sacroiliac joints and the sedimentation rate is raised. With pyogenic infections, the patient may be febrile, but there is very little else to define the nature of the underlying lesion. The damage to the sacroiliac joint may not be apparent for several weeks, and it is understandable that definitive diagnosis may, therefore, be delayed for a long period of time. If the clinician is very suspicious of the diagnosis, then a technetium scan may demonstrate a "hot spot" and the associated bony changes can then be defined by tomography. It must be remembered, however, that this area of the skeleton always takes up more technetium on a routine scan than other portions of the pelvis.

On occasion, a fluctuant abscess will form. Under such circumstances confirmation of the diagnosis and isolation of the organism can be achieved by needle biopsy. If aspiration proves impossible, then with the presumptive diagnosis provided by the overall clinical picture, the technetium scan, and tomography, open biopsy is mandatory in order that appropriate antibiotic therapy can be instituted.

Ewing's sarcomata have a predilection for the pelvis and when occurring adjacent to the sacroiliac joint may mimic the radiological appearance of destructive pyogenic arthritis. On occasion the differentiation from septic arthritis in such instances can only be established by open biopsy.

Because of the rarity of septic arthritis of the sacroiliac joint as a cause of backache and because of the nonspecific nature of the clinical picture, the diagnosis may easily be missed.

In summary, the patient does not look well and complains of pain in the sacroiliac region with tenderness on palpation. He is febrile and usually presents an elevated sedimentation rate and, in instances of pyogenic arthritis, an elevated white count. The x-rays may not show significant abnormality initially but continued concern over the possibility of the diagnosis should prompt the request for a technetium scan and tomography.

Summary

Affections of the sacroiliac region may present as backache. The anatomical characteristics of the joint and the natural history of ankylosis should prevent the occurrence of the so-called sacroiliac sprains.

Pelvic instability is an infrequent but definite hazard of taking a bone graft from the posterior superior iliac crest and is related to the inadvertent division of the iliolumbar ligament.

The introduction of the use of the histocompatibility antigen studies may lead to a redefinition of ankylosing spondylitis as a broader disease process. At present, x-ray changes in the sacroiliac joints are essential to a firm diagnosis.

The sophistication of a technetium scan minimizes the delays in diagnosis so prevalent with infections and neoplasms involving the sacroiliac region.

CHAPTER 6

Spondylogenic Backache:
Soft Tissue Lesions

"Knowledge of structure of the human body is the foundation on which all rational medicine and surgery is built."
—Mondini de Luzzi

The major factor that has clouded and confused the diagnosis of soft tissue lesions of the back is the phenomenon of referred pain. When a deep structure is irritated, either by trauma, disease, or by the experimental injection of an irritating solution, the pain resulting may be experienced locally, referred distally, or experienced both locally and radiating to a distance. It is important to recognize that tenderness may also be referred to a distance. The injection of hypertonic saline into the lumbosacral supraspinous ligament may give rise to pain radiating down the leg as far as the calf, and may also be associated with tender points commonly situated over the sacroiliac joint and the upper outer quadrant of the buttock (fig. 6.1).

The complaint of pain and the demonstration of local tenderness may obscure the fact that the offending pathological lesion is centrally placed and may lead the clinician to believe erroneously that the disease process underlies the site of the patient's complaints. This erroneous belief may apparently be confirmed by the temporary relief of pain on injection of local anesthetic. These points must be borne in mind when considering soft tissue lesions giving rise to low back pain.

MYOFASCIAL SPRAINS OR STRAINS

Partial tears of the attachment of muscles may occur, giving rise to local tenderness and pain of short duration. There is always a history of specific injury. The pain and tenderness are always away from the midline. This is a young man's injury with strong muscles guarding a healthy spine. A similar injury sustained by an older man, with weaker muscles and with degenerate discs, is much more likely to result in a posterior joint strain.

The lesions heal with the passage of time despite, rather than because of, treatment.

Injections of local anesthetic (with or without the addition of local steroids) into the areas of maximal tenderness certainly afford temporary relief of varying duration, but it is doubtful if they speed the resolution of the underlying pathology.

The symptoms may persist for about 3 weeks, during which time the patient is well advised to avoid provocative activity. If symptoms persist

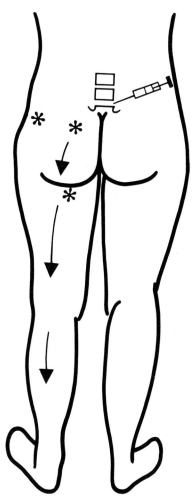

Fig. 6.1. The injection of hypertonic saline into the supraspinous ligament between L5 and S1 will give rise to local pain and pain referred down the back of the leg in sciatic distribution. In addition to this, there will be areas of tenderness produced in the lower limb most commonly at the sites noted by the asterisks.

beyond this period of time, then the problem should be carefully reassessed lest some more significant underlying lesion has been over-looked.

FIBROSITIS

The name "fibrositis" was first introduced by Sir William Gowers in 1904, when he coined the word to denote nonspecific inflammatory changes in fibrous tissue which he felt were responsible for the clinical syndrome of "lumbago." To date, the underlying pathological lesion has never been demonstrated histologically and it probably does not exist.

The so-called "fibrositic" nodules palpable over the iliac crest are usually localized nodules of fat. These anatomical variants are common. However, because they are situated in an area which is a common site of referred tenderness derived from a spinal lesion, they may be tender on pressure. The demonstration of a tender nodule associated with back pain and the occasional relief of symptoms by the injection of local anesthetic has lent weight to this clinical concept. Surgical exploration of the nodules revealed their true anatomical nature.

The concept of fibrositis ruling supreme as the most common cause of back pain for nearly half a century is a classic example of how the phenomenon of referred pain and tenderness has clouded the recognition of the pathological basis of low back pain derived from soft tissue disorders.

There is no reason why the term should not be retained to describe the clinical syndrome—*"low back pain of undetermined origin associated with tender nodules."* However, it must be remembered that the term does not denote a specific pathological process.

TENDINITIS

"Tendinitis" is again a clinical syndrome. The pathological basis of the lesion is inadequately defined. Clinically, it is recognized that very well localized areas of tenderness may develop at the attachment of tendons or ligaments to bone anywhere in the body and that these lesions are associated with a diffusely spreading pain. In the spine, breakdown changes of this nature may occur at the attachment of muscles to the sacrum or iliac crests or in the supraspinous ligaments and may give rise to a diffuse backache only vaguely related to activity. On examination, the area of breakdown presents a very small, but very well localized, area of tenderness. Pressure over the area not only elicits tenderness, but when maintained will reproduce the patient's symptoms.

The pathological basis of this syndrome is probably a local area of tendon breakdown or degeneration, which invokes an inflammatory or autoimmune response. It is possibly the vascular reaction, associated with localized edema, that accounts for the pain and tenderness. Empirically it has been found that gratifyingly rapid relief of pain can be obtained by the injection of steroids.

KISSING SPINES: SPRUNG BACK

Approximation of the spinous processes ("kissing spines") and the development of a bursa between them has been indicted as a cause of low back pain. "Sprung back" is a term coined by Newman to describe rupture of the supraspinous ligament following a sudden flexion strain applied to the spine with the pelvis fixed, as in falling on the buttocks with the legs out straight. It is doubtful whether either of these entities are, of themselves, a cause of low back pain (fig. 6.2).

With a normal disc, extension of a segment is limited by the anterior fibers of the annulus and at the limit of normal extension the spinous processes do not come into contact. Contact between the spinous processes is only seen with the abnormal mobility associated with disc degeneration. Although apposition of the spinous processes and the development of a painful bursitis may aggravate and intensify the symptoms derived from segmental instability associated with degenerative disc disease, it is never the sole source of symptoms. Following

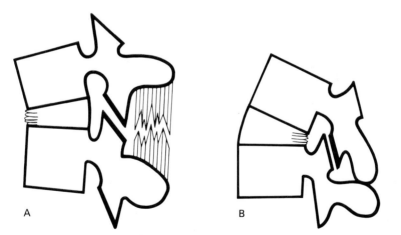

Fig. 6.2. *A*, An acute flexion injury of the spine may produce a tear of the supraspinous ligament. This lesion has been referred to as a "sprung back." It is unlikely, however, that this lesion can occur in the absence of gross disc degeneration which, by itself, is probably the source of the patient's complaints.

B, The radiological demonstration of apposition of the spinous processes has been referred to as "kissing spines." This anatomical disposition of the spinous processes cannot occur in the absence of an unstable disc segment. In the balance of probabilities, it is the associated disc degeneration rather than the bony apposition of the spinous processes that is the cause of the patient's symptoms.

partial or total excision of the spinous process in the treatment of this lesion, the basic underlying pathological defect of segmental instability still continues and remains productive of symptoms.

Forward flexion of the spine is limited by the posterior fibers of the annulus and the limit of forward flexion is achieved before there is any significant strain on the fibers of the supraspinous ligament. Surgical excision of a spinous process for biopsy, although it is inevitably associated with disruption of the supraspinous ligament, does not lead subsequently to the development of low back pain. Tearing of the supraspinous ligament can only occur in the presence of disc degeneration allowing an abnormal degree of flexion or with an injury severe enough to disrupt the posterior fibers of the annulus and the capsule of the posterior joints.

Separation and apposition of the spinous processes, when symptomatic, are indications of segmental instability associated with disc degeneration, and the treatment of such lesions, therefore, is the treatment of the associated disc degeneration.

DISC DEGENERATION

In order to understand the pathogenesis of symptoms derived from degenerative disc disease, it is necessary to have a clear concept of the mechanical changes that may arise from breakdown of an intervertebral disc.

The functional components of the intervertebral disc are described in chapter 1 where it is indicated that the combination of the annulus, the nucleus pulposus, and the hyaline cartilage plate makes for a very efficient coupling unit, provided all the structures remain intact. Once degenerative changes involve any one of the components of the disc, such as inspissation of the nucleus pulposus, a tear in the annulus, or a rupture of the hyaline cartilage plate, the smooth roller action is lost and the movement between adjacent vertebral segments becomes uneven, excessive, and irregular.

This is the stage of segmental instability. Excessive degrees of flexion and extension are permitted and a certain amount of backward and forward gliding movements occur as well. Normally, on flexion of the spine the discal borders of the vertebral bodies become parallel above the level of L5. This is the maximal movement permitted. In the stage of segmental instability, excessive degrees of extension and flexion are permitted and a certain amount of backward and forward gliding movement occurs as well (fig. 6.3).

This abnormal type of movement can be shown clinically by x-rays taken with the patients holding their spines in full extension and in full flexion. One problem posed by motion studies is the fact that, when a

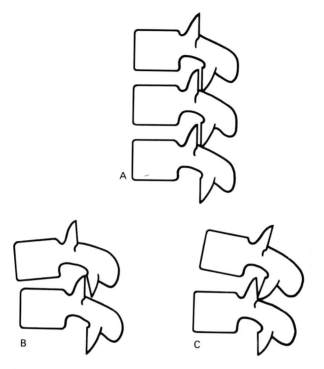

Fig. 6.3. In the early stages of degenerative disc disease, excessive degrees of flexion and extension are permitted at the involved segment. This abnormal mobility is associated with rocking of the posterior joints (*B* and *C*).

patient is in pain, the associated muscle guarding does not permit adequate flexion and extension x-rays to be taken. However, there are two radiological changes that are indicative of instability, the Knuttson phenomenon of air in the disc and the "traction spur."

The traction spur differs anatomically and radiologically from other spondylophytes in that it projects horizontally and develops about 2 mm above the vertebral body edge (fig. 6.4). It owes its development to the manner of attachment of the annulus fibers. In chapter 1 the mode of attachment of the outermost fibers to the undersurface of the epiphysial ring is described. With abnormal movements, an excessive strain is applied to these outermost fibers and it is here that the traction spur develops. It is the small traction spur that is clinically significant in that it is probably indicative of present instability. The large traction spur merely indicates that this segment has been unstable at some time in the past, but may be stable now, because of fibrotic changes occurring within the disc.

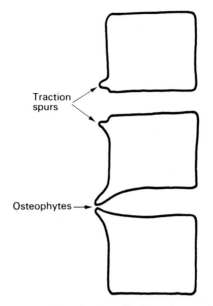

Traction spurs

Osteophytes →

Fig. 6.4. The traction spur projects horizontally from the vertebral body about 1 mm away from the discal border.

Segmental instability by itself is probably not painful, but the spine is vulnerable to trauma. A forced and unguarded movement may be concentrated on the wobbly segment and produce a posterior joint strain or a posterior joint subluxation. Repeated injuries may indeed produce osteochondral fractures and loose bodies in the posterior joints.

The next stage of disc degeneration is segmental hyperextension. Extension of the lumbar spine is limited by the anterior fibers of the annulus. When degenerative changes cause these fibers to lose their elasticity, the involved segment or segments may hyperextend (fig. 6.5).

A similar change may be seen in the next stage of disc degeneration, disc narrowing. As the intervertebral discs lose height, the posterior joints must override and subluxate (fig. 6.6). In both segmental hyperextension and disc narrowing, the related posterior joints in normal posture are held in hyperextension, and this postural defect is exaggerated if the patient has weak abdominal muscles and/or tight tensors, is overweight, is overwrought, and wears high heels—the typical North American housewife after four pregnancies.

When the posterior joints are held at the extreme of their limit of extension, there is no safety factor of movement and the extension strains of everyday living may push the joints past their physiologically permitted limits and thereby produce pain. Eventually the posterior joints may subluxate.

Repeated damage to the posterior joints, especially when associated with subluxation, will lead to degenerative changes. This is true osteoarthritis of the spine. Gross lipping of the vertebral bodies, often erroneously referred to as osteoarthritis of the spine, is merely a manifestation of disc degeneration (Fig. 6.7). Gross lipping may be present without associated degenerative changes in the posterior joints.

So much for the morbid anatomical changes associated with disc degeneration. What is the relationship of these changes to the pain experienced? In attempting to answer this, some clinical observations must be noted.

Scoliosis rarely gives rise to significant back pain even if left untreated, yet the lesion is associated with very gross posterior joint subluxation at many levels. The exception to this rule is the idiopathic lumbar scoliosis.

On the premise that the majority of backaches occur before the age of 40, the x-rays of 300 laborers, 40 years old, who had been engaged in heavy work all their lives, were reviewed. Of these, 150 denied any history of low back pain and 150 were under treatment for backache at the time of the review. A careful statistical analysis of the x-rays showed no difference in the incidence of anatomical variants and in the incidence of

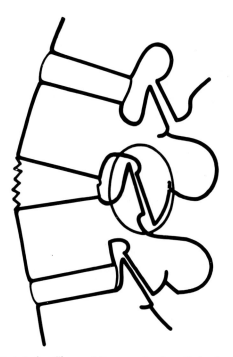

Fig. 6.5. When the anterior fibers of the annulus lose their elasticity, the involved segment falls into hyperextension permitting subluxation of the related posterior joint.

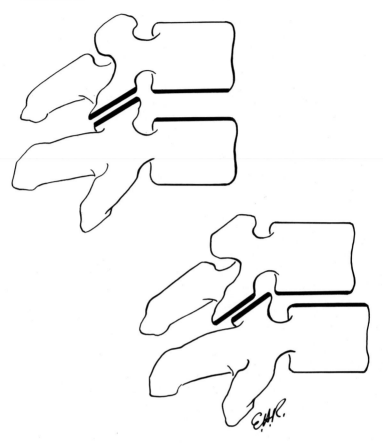

Fig. 6.6. As the intervertebral discs lose height and the vertebral bodies approach one another, the posterior joints must override and assume the position normally held in hyperextension. It is to be noted that owing to the inclination of the posterior joints, as the upper vertebral body approaches the vertebral body beneath it, it is displaced backwards producing a retrospondylolisthesis. This posterior displacement of the vertebral body, indicative of posterior joint subluxation, is readily recognizable on routine x-ray examination of the lumbar spine.

degenerative changes in the two groups studied. Indeed, some of the patients who had been employed in strenuous occupations all their lives without a twinge of back pain showed very marked degenerative changes on x-ray.

If every radiological sign of disc degeneration is given a numerical rating and these numbers are added together to give an arbitrary "degenerative index," it can be shown that, although radiological evidence of degenerative disc disease shows a linear increase with advancing years, the incidence of backache has a peak at 45 and thereafter tends to decline (fig. 6.8).

A patient may be seen with severe low back pain, and x-rays taken may show evidence of disc degeneration with segmental instability and posterior joint subluxation. After a period of conservative therapy, his

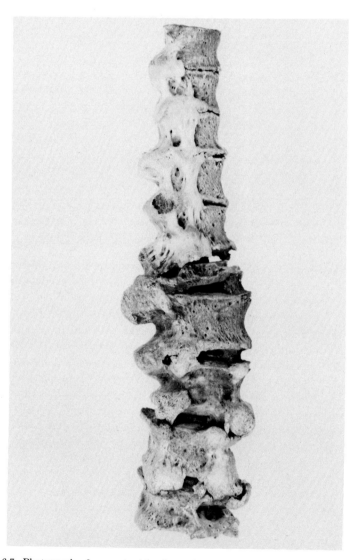

Fig. 6.7. Photograph of an excised lumbar spine showing the various bony outgrowths that are associated with disc degeneration. These bony outgrowths are correctly referred to as "spondylophytes."

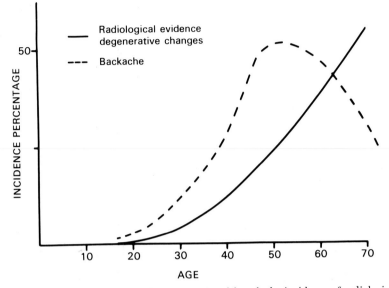

Fig. 6.8. It is to be noted from this graph that although the incidence of radiologically demonstrable degenerative changes in the lumbar spine increases with age, the maximal incidence of backache has a peak at 45 and thereafter tends to decline.

pain subsides and he returns to heavy work. Follow-up x-rays show identical changes even though the patient is completely symptom-free.

These observations and many similar instances must make the clinician question the significance of x-ray evidence of disc degeneration. On the other hand, it has been the experience of many that a patient previously incapacitated by low back pain, with radiological evidence of mechanical insufficiency of the spine due to disc degeneration, can, following a successful spinal fusion, return to strenuous activities without pain. In such instances surely mechanical instability was the cause of the original disability.

In our present stage of knowledge only the following may be stated: (1) disc degeneration may occur and may remain asymptomatic; (2) disc degeneration may be associated with changes *within the disc itself* which may be productive of pain; and (3) disc degeneration may give rise to mechanical instability which renders the spine vulnerable to trauma, as a result of which, pain may arise from ligamentous or posterior joint damage.

The pain experienced may remain localized to the back or there may be both local pain and referred pain or referred pain only. The experimental injection of hypertonic saline into the supraspinous ligament between D12 and L1 may give rise to pain referred to the low back and both buttocks and as low as the great trochanter. A similar injection into the supraspinous ligament between L5 and S1 may give rise to buttock pain and pain referred down the leg. The pain referred down the leg in sciatic distribution rarely goes below the knee, although on occasion it may extend to the ankle. Patients suffering from degenerative changes at the lumbodorsal or lumbosacral junction may present with pain referred in similar manner.

Posterior joint damage produced by degenerative changes of the L4-L5 disc may also produce pain referred to the groin. It is important to emphasize the fact that *pain down the leg associated with degenerative disc disease may indeed be referred pain and the patient's complaint of "sciatica" does not necessarily mean that a nerve root is being compromised.*

Degenerative disc disease may lead to nerve root compression under the following circumstances: disc ruptures, bony root entrapment, ligamentous root entrapment, and adhesive radiculitis.

DISC RUPTURES

In 1934, Mixter and Barr suggested that sciatic pain could result from irritation of a lumbar nerve root by a prolapsed intervertebral disc. Although skeptically received at first, this concept soon became universally accepted and founded the "dynasty of the disc," during which time the complaint of sciatic pain tended to become uncritically equated with the diagnosis of disc herniation. Surgical exploration of patients with evidence of lumbar root irritation has revealed the fact that there are indeed several sources of nerve root compromise, of which a ruptured intervertebral disc is but one example.

The term "herniated disc" tends to be used so loosely now as to lose much of its clinical significance, and indeed, there have been profusion and confusion of terminology (table 6.1). Sometimes the operative note will state with disarming simplicity, "a disc was found." The height of absurdity was the introduction of the term "concealed disc" to describe a herniated disc which could not be demonstrated at operation. One can imagine the confusion that would result if the term "concealed appendix" was considered an adequate explanation of a negative laparotomy.

Table 6.1. Synonyms for "Herniated Disc"

Herniated disc	Protruding disc
Prolapsed disc	Bulging disc
Sequestrated disc	Ruptured disc
Soft disc	Extruded disc
Slipped disc	"Disc"

To avoid further confusion, therefore, it is perhaps advisable to define the pathological state implied by the term "disc rupture."

The exact mechanism of a disc rupture has not been demonstrated, but it is a common misconception that a disc rupture consists of a extrusion of nuclear material through an annular defect much like toothpaste exuding through a hole in the side of a toothpaste tube. Operative experience belies this impression. It is unusual at operation to find a disc herniation consisting solely of extravasated nuclear material exuding through a defect in the annulus. The protrusion, extrusion, or sequestration always consists of varying amounts of nucleus, annulus, and cartilage plate.

Disc ruptures can be defined as distortions of the normal anatomical configuration of the annulus. Two major anatomical lesions can be defined: disc protrusion and disc herniations.

Disc Protrusions

Normally the annulus fibrosus forms a smooth continuous ring confining the nucleus pulposus. On occasion, following degenerative changes, a portion of the annulus fibrosus may give way and a localized bulge occurs even though the annular fibers are still intact.

With disc collapse, the annulus circumferentially protrudes beyond the peripheral rim of the vertebral bodies. The appearance is as though the disc had been made of putty and the vertebral bodies had been compressed together, a disc with a "middle-aged spread."

In disc protrusions then, the distortion of the annulus may be a localized annular bulge or a diffuse annular bulge. In both instances, the annular fibers remain intact and at operation, when a square window is cut in the annulus, the nucleus does not spontaneously extrude (fig. 6.9).

Disc Herniations

Disruption of the annular fibers permits prolapse, extrusion, or sequestration of the nucleus. Following detachment of a segment of the cartilage plate and disruption of the posterior annulus fibers, a portion of the annulus may be displaced posteriorly. The nucleus follows the displaced segment, and some nuclear material may be forced through the break in the annular fibers. Three types can be recognized, depending on the mode of displacement of nuclear material.

Prolapsed Intervertebral Disc

The displaced nuclear material is confined solely by a few of the outermost fibers of the annulus. At operation, a discreet prominence of the annulus can be demonstrated, and when this is incised, nuclear material spontaneously exudes through the incision.

DISC PROTRUSIONS
(ANNULAR FIBRES INTACT)

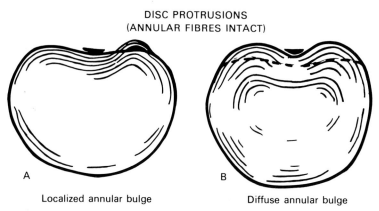

A   B

Localized annular bulge   Diffuse annular bulge

Fig. 6.9. In disc protrusions the annular fibers are not disrupted. The distortion of the normal configuration of the annulus may be confined to one side (a localized annular bulge) or the protrusion may be bilateral being constrained to some extent in the midline by the posterior longitudinal ligament.

Extruded Intervertebral Disc

In this lesion, the displaced nuclear material has burst through the posterior fibers of the annulus and lies under the posterior investing ligament. On incising this thin ligament, the extruded fragment can be recognized and picked up with forceps. As it is withdrawn from the wound, it can be seen that the tail of the fragment was lying in a defect in the annulus.

Sequestrated Intervertebral Disc

Nuclear material may be extruded through the posterior fibers of the annulus and through the posterior longitudinal ligament. The fragment lies free in the spinal canal. An extruded disc may therefore be associated with a sequestrated fragment which may remain trapped between the nerve root and the disc, or the free fragment may migrate. The sequestrated fragment may come to lie behind the vertebral body above or below the disc, in the axilla of the nerve root, in the intervertebral foramen, or in the midline anterior to the dural sac. On occasion, the freed portion of disc may erode or burst through the dura.

The sequestrated portion of the disc varies in size from a small fragment attached to the apex of the protrusion like a plume from an active valcano, to a massive segment of disc up to 20 ml in volume (fig. 6.10).

The Pathogenesis of Symptoms Resulting from Disc Ruptures

Some disc ruptures remain asymptomatic. Indeed, on routine screening of the lumbar spine when performing cervical myelography, 5% of

DISC HERNIATIONS
(ANNULAR FIBRES DISRUPTED)

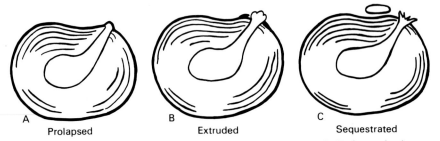

A   Prolapsed   B   Extruded   C   Sequestrated

Fig. 6.10. In disc herniations the annular fibers are disrupted. Under such circumstances the nucleus pulposus may be confined solely by the outermost fibers of the annulus
(prolapsed intervertebral disc); the nucleus may break through the outermost fibers of the
annulus and come to lie underneath the posterior longitudinal ligament (extruded
intervertebral disc); or a free fragment of nuclear material may break through the posterior
longitudinal ligament and lie free in the spinal canal (sequestrated intervertebral disc).

patients were shown to have a significant defect in the lumbar spine,
most frequently of the L4-L5 segment.

The method by which a disc rupture produces pain is not clear.
Physical pressure on a peripheral nerve does not produce pain; it
produces paresthesia. It is difficult then to understand why a common
symptom of disc herniation is indeed pain.

In examining this problem further, at the conclusion of a laminectomy,
a catheter was placed underneath the emerging nerve root of a segment
that had been decompressed and also underneath the normal nerve root
at the segment above. When the patients had recovered consciousness
and before they had been given any analgesics, the catheters were
distended. It was found that although distention of the catheter
underneath an involved, angry, red, inflamed nerve root reproduced the
sciatic pain, distention of the catheter underneath the normal nerve root
produced paresthesia only.

It is interesting to reflect that commonly in the early phases of a
disc herniation the patient may suffer from paresthesia only, giving rise
to an irritating, diffuse, ill-localized numbness in the lower leg and foot.
It would appear that the pain of a disc herniation is related to the
inflammatory reaction that occurs around the nerve root. The common
findings at operation are, of course, that the compressed nerve root looks
red, purplish, and angry and that this change is related to adventitious
tissue which has grown around the root and which contains new
nonmedullated, bare nerve endings of the type seen in granulation tissue
and of the type which seems sensitive to pressure, giving rise to a
sensation of pain.

Consideration of the mechanism of the pain resulting from a disc rupture is, of course, of importance when attempting to determine the mode of action of anti-inflammatory medication given systemically or anti-inflammatory agents such as hydrocortisone instilled around the nerve roots or in the epidural space.

The nerve roots in the cauda equina course obliquely over the intervertebral discs to emerge through the foramina of the vertebra below. Commonly, therefore, herniations of the lumbosacral disc will compromise the first sacral root (fig. 6.11), and a herniation of the disc between the fourth and fifth lumbar vertebrae will compress the fifth lumbar root (fig. 6.12). However, a lateral protrusion of the lumbosacral disc at the level of the foramen will distort the fifth lumbar root.

Compression of more than one root is seen under the following circumstances. A large herniation at the L5-S1 level may compromise both the first sacral root as it crosses over the disc and the fifth lumbar root as it emerges through the foramen (fig. 6.13). Similarly, a cranial, or more rarely a caudal migration of a sequestrated fragment may involve two roots. A massive central sequestration may involve several roots in the cauda equina with resulting bowel and bladder paralysis (fig. 6.14). This type of lesion is more commonly seen at the L4-L5 level than at any other level.

Unexpected root involvement is seen with prefixation or postfixation of the sciatic plexus. Bizarre clinical pictures may result from anomalies of root emergence as, for example, when both the fifth lumbar and first sacral roots emerge together through the lumbosacral canal (fig. 6.15).

Annular ruptures with disc herniations may occur on the lateral aspect of the disc, lateral to the intervertebral foramen, or the nerve root may be

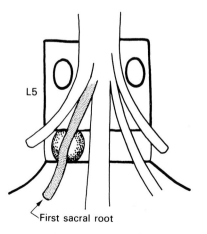

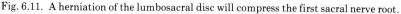

Fig. 6.11. A herniation of the lumbosacral disc will compress the first sacral nerve root.

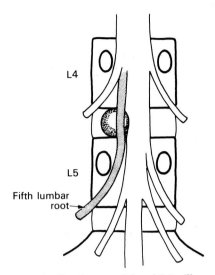

Fig. 6.12. A herniation of the disc between L4 and L5 will compress the fifth lumbar root.

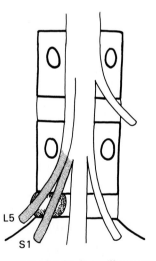

Fig. 6.13. A large herniation of the L5-S1 disc will compromise not only the nerve root crossing it, the first sacral nerve root, but also the nerve root emerging through the same foramen, the fifth lumbar nerve root.

engulfed by a diffuse bulge of the disc after it has emerged through the foramen (fig. 6.16). In both these instances the involved root is the root at the level of emergence. At the lumbosacral level, for example, with this type of lesion, it is the fifth lumbar root that is involved, not the first sacral, the usual victim of a lumbosacral disc herniation.

LIGAMENTOUS COMPRESSION

There is a strong ligamentous band which runs from the transverse process to the vertebral body. At the lumbosacral level the fifth root courses between this ligament and the ala of the sacrum (fig. 6.17). With disc collapse, the edge of the ligament descends on the nerve root and may trap it against the ala of the sacrum.

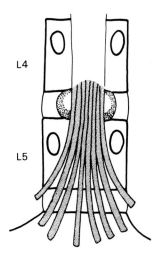

Fig. 6.14. A massive central sequestration of the disc at the L4-L5 level will involve all the nerve roots in the cauda equina and may result in bowel and bladder paralysis.

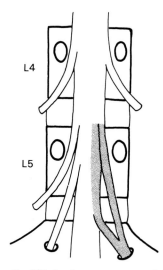

Fig. 6.15. In this diagram, the fifth lumbar nerve root and the first sacral nerve root are conjoined and emerge together through the first sacral foramen. A herniation of the lumbosacral disc will give rise to signs of first sacral and fifth lumbar root compromise.

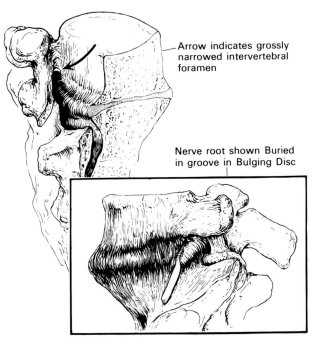

Arrow indicates grossly
narrowed intervertebral
foramen

Nerve root shown Buried
in groove in Bulging Disc

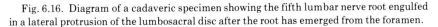

Fig. 6.16. Diagram of a cadaveric specimen showing the fifth lumbar nerve root engulfed in a lateral protrusion of the lumbosacral disc after the root has emerged from the foramen.

ADHESIVE RADICULITIS

This is a descriptive term rather than a pathological entity. In some forms of disc degeneration, the root becomes densely bound down to the back of the disc, and the histological autonomy of each rootlet is replaced by an almost malignantly invasive fibrotic reaction. Present experimental evidence would suggest that this is the result of an autoimmune response. The "tugging" on the tethered nerve root gives rise to a persistent, dull, nagging type of sciatic pain.

BONY ROOT ENTRAPMENT SYNDROMES

Narrowing of the spinal canal has been termed "spinal stenosis," and can be considered anatomically as being either lateral, giving rise to compression of the emerging nerve roots, or midline, resulting in compression of the cauda equina.

Bony compression of the emerging nerve roots arises as a result of subarticular entrapment, pedicular kinking, or foraminal impingement due to posterior joint subluxation.

Subarticular Entrapment

The nerve roots course downward and outward, passing underneath the medial border of the superior articular facets before they swing around the pedicle to emerge through the foramen. Hypertrophy of the superior articular facet may compress the nerve root between the facet and the dorsal aspect of the vertebral body (fig. 6.18).

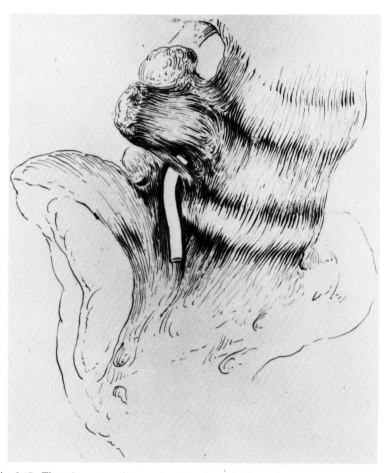

Fig. 6.17. There is a strong ligamentous band passing from the transverse process of L5 to the body of L5 which lies immediately cranial to the fifth lumbar nerve root as it courses over the ala of the sacrum. With marked narrowing of the lumbosacral disc, this ligament descends on the fifth lumbar nerve root like a guillotine and compresses it against the ala of the sacrum. Patients with this lesion will present with evidence of impairment of fifth lumbar nerve root function, but will not show any defect on myelographic examination.

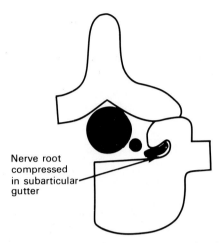

Fig. 6.18. The nerve root as it courses through the subarticular gutter may be compressed between a hypertrophied arthritic posterior joint and the dorsum of the vertebral body.

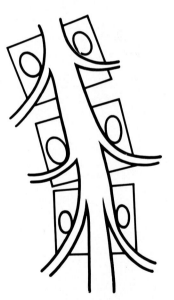

Fig. 6.19. With asymmetrical collapse of the disc and tilting of the vertebral body, the nerve root may be kinked by the pedicle giving rise to severe compression.

Pedicular Kinking

When advanced intervertebral disc degeneration is associated with marked narrowing of the disc, the vertebral bodies approach one another. As the upper vertebral body descends, its pedicle may, on occasion, kink the emerging nerve root to a significant degree if an asymmetrical collapse of the disc occurs (fig. 6.19). Commonly, however, the nerve root is seen to be compressed in a gutter formed by a diffuse lateral bulge of the disc and the pedicle above (fig. 6.20).

Foraminal Encroachment

As they emerge through the foramen, the nerve roots lie in close relation to the tip of the superior facet of the vertebra below. As the intervertebral disc narrows, the posterior joints override and the root may, on occasion, be compressed by the superior articular facet. Three different types of foraminal root compression are commonly seen (fig. 6.21).

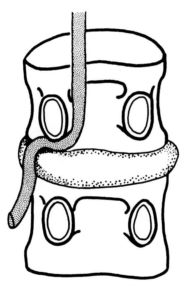

Fig. 6.20. In patients suffering from pedicular kinking of the nerve root, it is very common to find at operation that the nerve root is trapped in a gutter formed between a diffuse lateral bulge of the disc and the pedicle above.

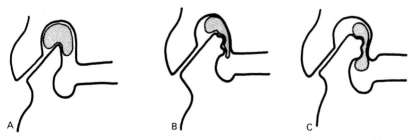

Fig 6.21. The nerve root may be trapped in the foramen. It may be compressed between the tip of a subluxated facet and the pedicle above (A); it may be compressed by osteophytic outgrowths on the superior articular facet (B); or it may be compressed between the facet and the dorsal aspect of the vertebral body (C).

Midline Compression

Midline compression may be a sequel of disc degeneration when, following narrowing of the intervertebral disc, the spinal canal is constricted by the presence of a diffuse annular bulge, anterior buckling of the ligamentum flavum, and shingling of the laminae posteriorly. This

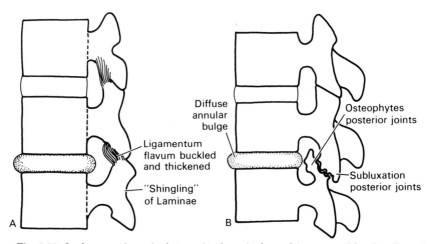

Fig. 6.22. In degenerative spinal stenosis, the spinal canal is narrowed by shingling of the laminae and by buckling of the ligamentum flavum. The arthritic posterior joints may hypertrophy and also encroach on the midline giving rise to further compression of the cauda equina. The emerging nerve roots are commonly compressed as they course through the narrow subarticular gutter.

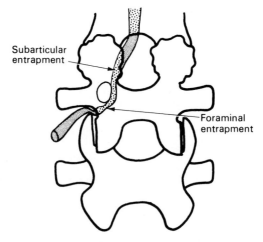

Fig. 6.23. In apophysial stenosis an emerging nerve root may be compressed at two sites. For example, as in this diagram, it may be compressed as it passes through the subarticular gutter and it may also be trapped in the foramen by the tip of the superior articular facet.

constraint may be further aggravated by overgrowth of the arthritic posterior joints which may indeed also encroach on the midline (fig. 6.22).

Forward displacement of the laminae seen in degenerative spondylolisthesis and the thickening of the lamina seen in certain pathological states such as fluoridosis and occasionally Paget's disease may produce a posterior encroachment of the spinal canal. Any technique of spinal fusion that involves decortication of the laminae with or without the addition of a bone graft may produce a diffuse hypertrophy of the posterior elements leading to constriction of the spinal canal. Postfusion spinal stenosis is, of course, more likely to occur if, prior to surgery, the patient was suffering either from a congenital narrowing of the spinal

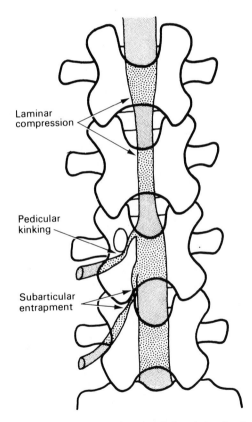

Laminar compression

Pedicular kinking

Subarticular entrapment

Fig. 6.24. Spinal stenosis must always be regarded as being laminar and apophysial. Laminar stenosis will compromise the cauda equina; apophysial stenosis will compromise the emerging nerve roots. It is important to recognize, however, as shown in this diagram, that the midline compression may occur at a different level from the apophysial compression of the emerging nerve roots.

canal or a narrowing produced by degenerative changes of the type previously described.

Various combinations and permutations of laminar and apophysial compression are seen. For example, the fifth lumbar nerve root may be compressed as it courses under the superior articular facet at L5, and it may also be trapped in the foramen by the tip of the superior articular facet of S1 (fig. 6.23). Although laminar compression at times may occur by itself, it is frequently associated with lateral or apophysial root entrapment which may arise at the same segment or the laminar and apophysial compressions may be at different segments (fig. 6.24).

Spinal stenosis then may be defined as narrowing of the spinal canal. This narrowing may be apophysial and may compress the nerve roots at their point of emergence at one or more segments. The compression may be midline and produced by the laminae or it may be a result of a combination of both these mechanisms, at the same level, or at different segments.

Midline compression of the cauda equina may produce backache only. Clinical evaluation of patients has suggested that radicular pain commonly implies lateral compression or root stenosis. Unlike the radicular pain of disc herniations, the sciatic pain frequently presents a claudicant character. In contradistinction to intermittent claudication of vascular insufficiency, the pain is more commonly experienced in the thigh than in the calf and, although the symptoms may become progressively more severe with walking, as they do with vascular insufficiency, the pain does not abate on standing still. The patient has to sit down or lie down to obtain relief. Some patients experience increasing subjective weakness on continuing to walk, and on occasion an increase in objective evidence of impairment of root conduction may be demonstrated on examination.

CHAPTER 7

The History

"A doctor who cannot take a good history and a patient who cannot give one are in danger of giving and receiving bad treatment."

Anonymous

When taking an adequate history, patience is not only a virtue, it is a vital necessity as the following verbatim report of the first part of a prolonged consultation reveals:

Doctor:

"Well, Mrs. Jones, what can I do to help you today?"

Patient:

"I sure hope you can cure it."

D:

"Well, I'll try. Have you any pain?"

P:

"Of course I have, I wouldn't be here if I didn't have any pain. I'm not the sort of person that keeps running to doctors with nothing wrong with them. I know you're all very busy and if . . . "

D:

"Where is the pain?"

P:

"The same place it's always been."

D:

"Where is that?"

P:

"In my back, of course."

D:

"Where about in your back, in the low back?"

P:

"I don't know whether you would call it low or high. All I can say is it's sure a bad pain."

D:

"Could you point to the pain. Ah, I see. How long have you had this?"

P:

"Ever since I tripped on the stairs."

D:

"When was that?"

P:

"Didn't my doctor send you my history? His nurse promised me faithfully she'd post them to you. Oh, this is terrible. I don't see any point in my coming here if you don't know anything about me. I wonder why . . . "

D:

"When did you have the accident on the stairs?"

P:

"In June."

D:

"Have you had pain everyday since then?"

P:

"Sometimes."

D:

"You mean the pain is intermittent?"

P:

"No. I mean sometimes I have the pain and sometimes I don't."

D:

"When you have the pain what aggravates it?"

P:

"How do you mean aggravates?"

D:

"Does anything make the pain worse?"

P:

"No, it's worse all the time."

D:

"Does lifting make the pain more severe?"

P:

"No."

D:

"You can lift anything you want without hurting your back?"

P:

"No, I can't lift nothing."

D:

"Why?"

P:

"Because of my back."

D:

"Let's just think of some of the things you do in your house. Does

vacuum cleaning, bed making, doing the laundry—do any of these
things make it worse?"

P:

"If I could do all those things I wouldn't be here. I don't believe in
running to the doctor with the least little thing. I can take a lot of
pain more than most people. You ask my husband. I can't even sit
down because of the pain."

D:

"Does anything relieve your back pain?"

P:

"No."

D:

"What do you do when the pain is bad?"

P:

"I lie down."

D:

"Does lying down make the pain better?"

P:

"No. It's just as bad when I get up."

D:

"When you are actually lying down is the pain any easier?"

P:

"Yes, but I can't spend my life lying down."

D:

"Does this pain stop you from doing anything you want to do?"

P:

"I can't play golf with my husband."

D:

"Do you get a lot of pain in your back everytime you play golf?"

P:

"Yes."

D:

"When did you last play golf?"

P:

"Eight years ago."

D:

"Why haven't you tried to play golf again?"

P:

"My doctor told me not to."

It is easy to describe a color, a sound, a taste, or a smell because these
are sensations that can be shared. "I went down to the beach later that
evening, when the setting sun had turned the sea into a vivid red and all

that could be heard was the plaintive cry of the seagulls and the gentle splashing of the waves against the rocks." Statements such as this make a clear impression in the mind of the listener. It is more difficult, and yet more important, to interpret the statement "I have this uncomfortable feeling in my back—I wouldn't call it a pain really," or "I was paralyzed with pain that felt like red hot rivers rushing down my legs." Is the second patient exaggerating, or has he got more serious trouble in his back?

When taking a history it is not good enough to find out that the patient has "back pain" or that he has pain in his right leg or left leg. It is essential to obtain a description of the pain in meticulous detail. Having obtained a clear description of the discomforts the patient is suffering from, it is then necessary to find out as much as you can about the personality of the patient and his activities in order to try to correlate the pain to the disability about which the patient is complaining. The majority of patients don't come because of pain: they come because of the disability it produces. "I've got this backache and I can't play badminton." He can do everything else; he wants you to overcome his "disability" and make him able to play badminton again.

> You have to obtain a clear picture of the pain.

> From this you must assess the possible source of pain.

> You have to obtain an equally clear picture of the patient who has the pain.

> From these facts you have to assess why the pain is causing the complained of disability.

The Picture of the Pain

The Site of the Pain

When a patient states he has "back pain," he may mean anywhere from the base of the neck to the buttocks. It is not good enough to ask the patient where he feels the pain; he must demonstrate it. A patient's grasp of anatomy is understandably vague. When a patient says that he has pain in his back, he may be referring to the interscapular region in his back, and even when he states that he has pain in the "small of the back" he may be referring to the lumbodorsal junction. When a patient describes pain in the "hip," he generally means pain in the buttock. It is necessary always to get the patient to point to where he has the pain.

The method the patient chooses to demonstrate the site of pain is instructive. The emotionally stable patient generally places the palm of the hand at the site of maximal pain and moves it across his body to demonstrate the route of radiation. The psychologically destroyed patient generally points out the area of his pain with his thumb (fig. 7.1). He never touches the painful area. The pain, so to speak, is outside his soma.

Spread of pain to the leg is an important symptom and the patients should be asked to demonstrate the distribution of the pain. To a patient, a leg is a leg, and most will not volunteer any information as to whether the pain is in the front of the thigh or at the back of the thigh, whether it radiates down to the knee, or whether it goes below the knee. It is important to know this when trying to determine whether the patient

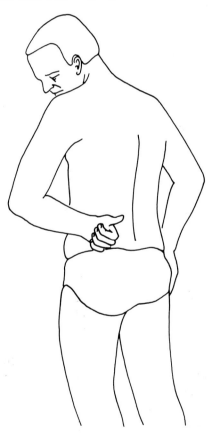

Fig. 7.1. Patients who are suffering from a significant emotional overlay will frequently point to the area of pain in the lower back with their thumb. They never actually touch their body.

is suffering from referred pain or whether the pain in the leg is due to root irritation and, if so, which root.

Referred pain is rarely felt below the knee, whereas pain due to root irritation may spread to the calf or even into the foot. Pain resulting from compression of the fourth lumbar root usually radiates down the front of the thigh.

Pain due to root irritation is frequently associated with paresthesia or a sensation of numbness. Paresthesia involving the lateral border of the foot may be associated with an S1 lesion, but a patient with an L5 lesion may describe numbness over the dorsum of the foot and even in the big toe.

The presence of these symptoms is helpful in making the diagnosis of root irritation and localizing the level of involvement. The patient does not usually volunteer this information; it must be asked for specifically.

Influence of Activities

Specific questions must be asked to determine the factors that influence the pain. Backache due to a mechanical breakdown of the spine is almost always aggravated by general and specific activities and is relieved by rest. There are, of course, some exceptions to this general rule, but on the whole it is fairly reliable. Backache due to a penetrating duodenal ulcer is not aggravated by activities, nor does it ease if the patient lies down. Patients with a neurofibroma involving a nerve root frequently give a history of having to get up at night to walk around to "get away" from the pain and patients with a secondary deposit in the spine commonly give the story of sudden cramps of pain in their back even when lying down. A few patients with disc degeneration find that their pain is worse lying in bed, but this is most unusual. Patients who complain of pain in bed may sleep face downward, a position which, by extending the lumbar spine, aggravates discogenic pain. Constant pain in bed is also seen in the emotionally distraught.

When trying to find out whether activities increase the pain, it is best to ask specific questions. "Does lifting hurt?" "Is your pain worse when you bend over the washbasin?" "Can you make beds?" "Can you use the vacuum cleaner?" "Is the pain made worse by walking or climbing stairs?" Discogenic pain is frequently increased by maintaining one posture over a period of time: prolonged walking, prolonged sitting, or prolonged standing. Sudden jars will aggravate any form of mechanical pain. The history of pain shooting down the leg as a result of coughing or sneezing is highly suggestive of root compression.

Many patients are confused by the question, "Is your pain better when you lie down?" They will frequently answer, "No," in the belief that the question implied that the act of lying down completely cured their backache for some time. They may answer "No, it is not made better by lying down; it is just as bad as ever when I get up." It is probably better to ask them, "What do you feel like doing when the pain is very bad?" Although some patients may regard this question as being absurd, most will tell you they would like to lie down, or sit down, if they could.

Although it may be tedious at times, it is imperative to learn from the patient what aggravates and what relieves his symptoms.

Duration and Progression of Symptoms

It is important to have a clear knowledge of the onset, duration, and progression of the symptoms. How did the pain start? Gradually or suddenly? Did it follow provocative activity? Has the pain been continuous or intermittent?

The sudden onset of pain following provocative activity with an intermittent course subsequently is highly suggestive of a mechanical basis for the symptoms.

Is the pain getting worse? If the patient feels that his symptoms are getting progressively worse, is this because the attacks are more frequent, more severe, and more prolonged, or is it because the patient has lost all his tolerance and is fed up with this bothersome burden?

The Anatomical Basis of the Pain

It must be remembered that back pain is a symptom and not a disease and that its source may lie outside the spine. It is essential, therefore, to include in the history a general functional enquiry. For example, the history of dorsolumbar pain relieved by the ingestion of food raises the possibility of a penetrating duodenal ulcer. The history of difficulty in micturition demands further enquiry to rule out prostatic cancer with secondaries in the spine. A family history of diabetes raises the possibility of a diabetic neuritis. A diabetic diathesis, by itself, markedly intensifies the pain of root compression. A chronic cough or a history of unexplained weight loss cannot be ignored.

It cannot be overemphasized that a spondylogenic back pain is aggravated by general and specific activities and is relieved, to some extent, by recumbency.

The Patient

Emotional Responses

Emotional responses play a large role in the disability associated with low back pain and these will become evident as the patient tells his story. It must always be remembered that emotional breakdowns do not protect a patient against organic disease; they merely make the diagnosis and treatment more difficult. Without discussing esoteric psychological phenomenon—without any attempt at following acceptable psychological terminology—I shall describe five common syndromes frequently seen in clinical practice: the racehorse syndrome, the razor's edge syndrome, the worried-sick syndrome, the last straw factor, and the camouflaged emotional breakdown.

The Racehorse Syndrome. The racehorse syndrome applies to the group of tense, hard driving, hyper-reactive patients. Under stressful situations they tend to hyperextend their backs and assume the fight position. Throughout their lives they have responded to tense situations in this manner without pain. However, once they develop disc degeneration, the segmental instability allows the related posterior joints to be pushed beyond the permitted physiological range when this posture is adopted, and pain results. The pain that they experience interferes with their ability to get on with their normal way of life, and the frustration that they feel increases the tension in their sacrospinales, thereby, aggravating and perpetuating their discomforts. In the treatment of these patients, the significance of this postural change must be explained. In addition to the routine conservative treatment of discogenic back pain, they should be taught voluntary muscle relaxation, and they need mild sedation to take the edge off their normal tensions and anxieties.

The Razor's Edge Syndrome. The razor's edge syndrome refers to patients who precariously tread their way through life on the razor's edge of emotional stability. These patients with hysterical personalities, like people in show business, play their lives in high C.

Before the recent changes in sartorial habits, they could be spotted easily. The women loved outlandish hair styles and heavy eye make-up. They decorated themselves with large earrings and rows of necklaces. Multiple bracelets and bangles adorned their wrists, and they wore huge garish rings on their fingers. The men affected beards and dark glasses which they wore indoors. Although dress and hairstyle can no longer be regarded as being of diagnostic significance, the dramatization of symptoms is characteristic. Superlatives are thrown around with gay abandon. The pain is "agonizing." "I was paralyzed with pain." "It was as though someone was tearing the muscles out of my leg." " . . . like boiling water poured on my back." "I haven't had a wink of sleep in 2 months."

Examination reveals diverse corporal contortions such as twitching, turning, writhing and rolling about, and the examiner's discovery of tender points is invariably vocally acknowledged by wails, moans, groans, and sharp intakes of breath or uncontrolled and alarming shouts.

No drug will give these patients a chemical vacation from their exhausting reaction to life. If the underlying cause of their symptoms can be recognized through the emotional smoke screen they have put up, it should be treated along routine lines. When the cause of the pain has been overcome, they will return to a way of life that is normal for them.

Hysterical reactions are common in childhood. When a child grazes his knee he walks with a stiff leg. There is no need to do this; it is a hysterical response to injury—an exaggerated response for the purposes of gain, namely, attention and sympathy. In a child this is understood and tolerated with a smile. In an adult, the same response generally irritates the physician and indeed may irritate him to such a degree that examination tends to be superficial and treatment perfunctory. At times it is difficult to remember that these patients cannot control or modify their reactions—it is in their genes; they are built this way. The physician is treating a patient, not a spine, and regardless of the bizarre description of the symptoms and the histrionics on examination, he must accept the possibility of a physical disorder and investigate its probability in every instance.

The Worried-Sick Syndrome. Only a moron is totally unconcerned about the development of inexplicable symptoms. Most patients are concerned not only about the cause of their symptoms but also about their significance. Many have seen relatives in the terminal phases of malignancy whose last symptom was low back pain. Many associate pain in the back with "arthritis," and this fear may be reinforced by being told previously that the "x-rays of the spine showed arthritic changes . . . " To most patients arthritis denotes a relentlessly progressive dread disease leading eventually to confinement in a wheelchair. These fears are common, although not commonly expressed. Above all else, the physician must reassure the patient and disabuse him of unfounded anxieties. If the patient has disc degeneration, he must never be told he has "arthritis of the spine."

Anxiety may be a form of intelligent concern, but in some born to worry, an almost pathological unfounded concern about their symptoms may be more disabling than the pain itself. These patients confuse the words "hurting" and "harming." Every time they do something that increases pain, they are terrified they have done themselves irreparable damage. They treat their backs as though they are made of Dresden china, fearful of doing anything that may aggravate the lesion and thereby prolong their disability. Their problem may be compounded by their physician's advice. In the routine management of discogenic back pain, they may be told to avoid certain activities such as bending, lifting, playing tennis, or bowling. This is good advice, but they must also be told that these modifications of activity are suggested to decrease discomforts, not to prevent damage. Unless told this, the patients may gradually cut themselves out of all activities until eventually they just vegetate.

"This back pain is completely ruining my life—I can't bowl, I can't ski, I can't play golf, I can't do anything," the patient may say. "Do you get a lot of pain when you do these things?" "I don't know—I haven't done anything for 2 years." "Why haven't you tried to play a game of golf again?" "My doctor told me I shouldn't."

After weeks or months of inactivity, it will be extremely difficult to get these patients back to the business of normal living. Every increase in activity may be associated with a new twinge of pain which may frighten them back to the security of their beds. Their problems are compounded by apprehension and misapprehension, and the physician must deal firmly with both.

The hypochondriac can be regarded as another example of the "worried-sick syndrome." Everyone is wary of the patients who consult pages of notes, and the physician should be equally wary of the husband who brings his wife to substantiate his story. Never forget, however, that sometimes the hypochondriac is right.

The Last Straw Factor. The havoc wrought by a back pain on a patient's life may destroy the patient's emotional stability as, for example, the patient who speaks little English and who has no special skills, who works as a laborer in a small town, supporting a wife and five children. An insecure job situation, because of industrial recession in the area, keeps him constantly concerned about his ability to keep up payments on his debts. The back pain resulting from an accident stops him working for a few days. A recurrence without provocative trauma makes both the employer and the patient doubtful about his ability to hold down a job, and the third attack finds him unemployed. Inability to find alternative employment increases his debts and articles of furniture are repossessed by the finance company. To this patient, his backache is the major disaster of his life, and his symptoms and signs may well be exaggerated beyond recognition.

The patient cannot be helped solely by measures directed at his back. His whole problem has to be alleviated and the help of all social services has to be enlisted.

The Camouflaged Emotional Breakdown. Depressive states are common between the ages of 45 and 55. These patients, commonly very active when younger, find that as their psychic energy decreases, as they move into second gear, they are increasingly unable to cope with the demands made on them. Despite the term "depression," they do not present the picture of melancholia. They demonstrate concealed or overt hostility. They are more easily provoked to anger and tears. They are increasingly critical of the faults they recognize in the people around them. They are constantly tired and sleep does not refresh them. They do not sleep well and frequently awaken early in the morning. They can't make decisions. They don't want to go out and they hate staying in. They lose their sense of fun. They claim that this unsociable state is the result of their wretched spine. Remember, a persistent backache seldom makes people miserable, but miserable people frequently have backache and complain loudly about it.

The back pain from which they suffer becomes a scapegoat to explain their inability to cope with life. "I was always a very active woman. I was President of the local P.T.A., I was one of the campaign organizers for the last election, and I always went with my husband on his trips, but, with this backache, I am useless." They have an almost delusional belief in the organicity of their symptoms. They believe and would like you to believe that had it not been for the backache they would still be a leader in the community and, characteristically when giving the history, they will constantly refer back to this restriction in nonphysical activities.

The curtailment of their activities is not solely due to their backache. In better emotional health they could cope with their discomforts, mollifying and minimizing their pain with mild analgesics and a slight modification of their daily rounds. Simple therapeutic measures directed at the organic basis of these patients' complaints will not permit them to return to normal activities. Failure of conservative treatment may lead to desperation surgery, nearly always attended with poor results and an aggravated deterioration in the patient's emotional health. Treatment must be directed at the patient as a whole and psychiatric guidance must be sought early.

This is a very superficial reference to the infinite varieties of emotional responses that may modify the patient's reaction to pain in the back and may distort the history given. One cardinal principle must be remembered: there is no such thing as imaginary pain. Apart from the very rare occurrence of malingering, everyone has the pain that they say they have, but the emotional response to the pain will significantly influence the resulting disability. In the treatment of these patients, the physician must analyze the constitution of their disability, that is to say, how much of the disability is due to the emotional response. In the course of doing this, the physician must *never* give the impression that he thinks the patient is imagining his symptoms. "Inappropriate disability" and *total* lack of response to reasonable modalities of therapy are the first and most important clues that the physician will obtain to indicate that he is dealing with a patient destroyed by a psychogenic regional pain.

The Disability

With a clear picture of the pain the patient has and with an adequate impression of the patient who has the pain, it should be possible to assess the disability and its possible source.

Is the patient significantly disabled or do the symptoms just constitute an irritating nuisance or, indeed, is the "disability" just an understandable concern regarding the cause and significance of the pain?

Is the disability related to one aspect of the patient's life and is this significant? "I can't jog."

Does the disability interfere with the patient's capacity to do his work and his ability to enjoy himself in his leisure hours and, if so, to what extent?

Is the disability disproportionately extreme ("I haven't been able to get out of bed for 2 months") and, therefore, representative of a psychogenic regional pain or a psychogenic magnification of the symptoms derived from an underlying physical disorder?

In summary you are treating a patient and not a spine. In order to do this adequately, you must find out as much as you can about the patient who has the back pain as well as finding out as much as you can about the back pain the patient has.

CHAPTER 8

Examination of the Back

"More mistakes are made from want of proper examination than for any other reason."

—Russell Howard

"The examining physician often hesitates to make the necessary examination because it involves soiling the finger."

—William Mayo

The purpose of this chapter is to give a general outline of a routine clinical examination of a patient suffering from significant back pain. Specific findings are alluded to again when the examination and treatment of common clinical syndromes are discussed. It is important to emphasize that accurate records of the history and examination should be made. These must include exact measurements and not vague terms such as "good," "poor," "limited," etc. Good records are necessary for case analysis, for comparison and on case reviews, for assistance to a consulting physician, and, at times, for legal purposes.

The examination of the back should be conducted in an orderly predetermined manner. Examination of the patient should not be directed solely at eliciting signs of a specific disease suggested by the history, nor should individual systems be examined serially: neurological examination, abdominal examination, vascular examination, etc. The examination must be conducted in an orderly manner so that all possible physical findings may be evaluated. The first prerequisite is that the patient must be undressed. A cursory examination is worse than no examination at all because it may give the false hope that the lesion is minor.

Gross postural changes are first noted: hyperlordosis and the reverse, flattening of the back, associated with muscle spasm as seen in disc herniations and inflammatory lesions. Lateral curvatures are noted. The curve of an idiopathic scoliosis differs from the list of the spine associated with root compression in that sciatic scoliosis disappears on recumbency.

Structural scoliosis produces a razorback eminence of the thoracic cage. An advanced ankylosing spondylitis produces a fixed kyphosis. Local changes such as undue prominence of the spinous process of L5 in

117

spondylolisthesis and a sag of one buttock crease sometimes seen in an S1 root lesions should be noted at this stage of the examination. The first phase of the examination then is a thorough inspection of the back as a whole.

The range and rhythm of spinal movements are next tested. The range of forward flexion is recorded by noting how far the hands come toward the floor. The rhythm of forward flexion is observed by placing the finger-tips on the spinous processes and noting how far they separate on flexion of the spine (fig. 8.1).

Extension is recorded by noting how far the patient can lean backwards before the pelvis tilts. Lateral flexion is measured by noting how far the patient can slide his hand down his thigh toward his knee (fig. 8.2). Rota-

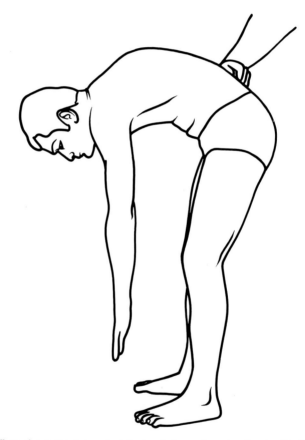

Fig. 8.1. When the patient is asked to bend forward, not only should the range of movement be noted, but the ability of the spinous processes to separate should also be recorded. This is best done by placing the finger tips over the spinous processes in the lumbar spine.

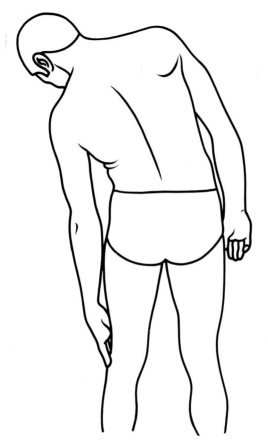

Fig. 8.2. Lateral flexion is recorded by noting how far the patient can slide his hand down his thigh toward his knee.

tion can be tested by getting the patient to stand with his feet wide apart and rotate with his hands on his hips (fig. 8.3).

During the examination, observe any specific abnormalities, for example, marked limitation of the range of forward flexion without lumbar movement, as in root irritation due to disc herniation. These patients frequently show deviation to the painful side on forward flexion. The rigidity of the whole spine in the later stages of ankylosing spondylitis is characteristic. Reversal of normal spinal rhythm on attempting to regain the erect posture after forward flexion is characteristic of disc degeneration associated with a posterior joint lesion. To avoid putting an extension strain on the posterior joints, the patient tucks his pelvis under his spine to regain the erect position. When getting up from forward flexion, he will start to extend the spine, but this movement is uncomfortable. To

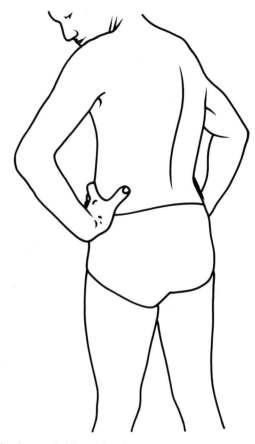

Fig. 8.3. Rotation is recorded by asking the patient to place his hands on his hips. The elbows then act as the arms of a goniometer and the degree of rotation permitted can be measured.

avoid this, he will slightly flex his hips and knees in order to tuck the pelvis under the spine and then regain the erect position by straightening the legs (fig. 8.4).

With the patient still standing, the strength of the gastrocnemius is determined by testing the ability to stand on tiptoe (fig. 8.5). Lesions involving the first sacral root such as lumbosacral disc herniation may produce weakness of tiptoe raising and diminution of the ankle jerk which can be tested with the patient kneeling on a chair. The examiner must remember that if a patient has a weak quadriceps his leg will tend to buckle on attempting to rise on tiptoe. This is a diagnostic trap for the unwary.

With the patient sitting on the edge of the bed, the knee jerks are tested. It must be emphasized that in the examination of the back an orderly scheme of examination must be followed to avoid missing any important findings.

The patient should next lie supine on the bed to allow reflexes to be tested and the power of the dorsiflexors of the ankles to be assessed. The dorsiflexors of the ankles may become weak with lesions involving the fifth lumbar nerve root such as herniation of the disc between the fourth and fifth lumbar vertebra. The medial hamstring reflex may also be diminished with compromise of the fifth lumbar root.

One feature of the plantar response is a reflex contraction of the tensor fascia femoris. This portion of the withdrawal response is lost with lesions involving S1.

The strength of the dorsiflexors should not be tested with the knee extended because if the patient has significant sciatic pain any attempt by the patient to resist forced plantar flexion of the ankle will be painful and a false impression of weakness may be obtained. The knee should be flexed and full body weight pressure applied against the dorsum of the foot to assess the strength of the dorsiflexors (figs. 8.6). Lesions involving the fifth lumbar root may cause weakness of the extensor haliucis

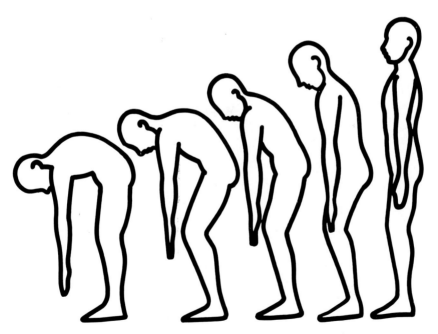

Fig. 8.4. Reversal of spinal rhythm. On attempting to regain the erect position from forward flexion, the patient will bend the knees and tuck the pelvis underneath the spine in order to stand erect. This type of movement is very characteristic of segmental instability.

longus before any significant weakness of the dorsiflexors of the ankle is apparent. Similarly, with an S1 lesion, flexor hallucis longus may become detectably weak before there is any noticeable weakness of the gastrocnemius. Sometimes this can be dramatically demonstrated by asking the patient to claw or flex his toes whereupon it may be noted that he can flex the big toe on one side but not on the other.

The quadriceps may be weak with lesions of the fourth lumbar nerve root. The strength of the muscle is best tested with the patient lying on his back with the hips slightly flexed and the knee placed over the examiner's forearm. The patient then tries to extend the knee against the resistance of the examiner's other hand.

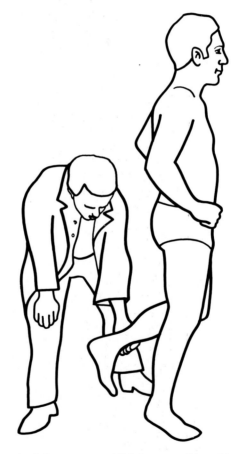

Fig. 8.5. The strength of the gastrocnemeii is best tested by asking the patient to rise on tiptoe repetitively and rapidly. You are looking for fatiguability and therefore the patient must be asked to rise on tiptoe a minimum of 10 times.

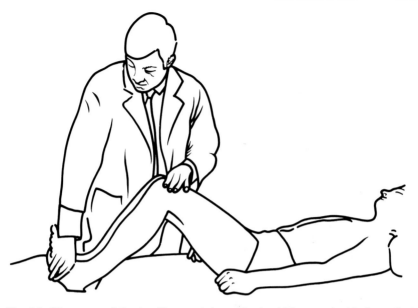

Fig. 8.6. The power of the dorsiflexors of the ankle should be tested with the patient lying on his back with his hips and knees flexed. The patient holds his ankle in full dorsiflexion and attempts to resist the maximal force that the physician can apply to the dorsum of the foot.

Diffuse weakness of all muscle groups, particularly the psoas, is highly suggestive of an emotional breakdown. Functional or emotional weakness is characterized by jerky relaxation of the muscles regardless of what force is applied. Quite frequently these patients will be able to resist breakdown of a fixed position, but will be unable to initiate movement of a joint against weak resistance. This is the so-called discrepant motor weakness. In gross emotional disturbances, there may be diffuse unreasonable weakness of many muscle groups. Characteristically these patients will be unable to extend the terminal interphalangeal joint of the thumb against the slightest resistance and will not be able to hold their eyes closed tightly shut when the examiner tries to push the eyebrow up.

Nerve root irritation is commonly associated with specific muscle tenderness. With first sacral root irritation the calf becomes tender. With fifth lumbar root irritation the anterior tibial muscles become tender, and with fourth lumbar root irritation the quadriceps are tender. Tenderness over the subcutaneous surface of the tibia is seen when emotional overtones play a large part in the clinical picture. Specific muscle tenderness is a very important physical sign of root irritation.

With the patient still supine, appreciation of pinprick can be tested, comparing the sensibility of the same areas in both legs. Dermatome

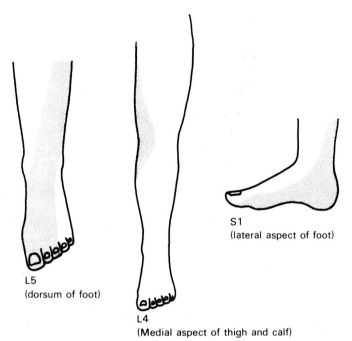

L5
(dorsum of foot)

S1
(lateral aspect of foot)

L4
(Medial aspect of thigh and calf)

Fig. 8.7. Although areas of sensory innervation can be variable, commonly the first sacral root supplies the sole and the lateral border of the foot. The area of skin just behind the lateral malleolus is an autonomous area for the first sacral root.

The fifth lumbar root supplies the dorsum of the foot and the anterior aspect of the lower leg. The autonomous area for the fifth lumbar root is the skin over the first interdigital cleft.

The fourth lumbar root supplies the anteromedial aspect of the thigh.

areas are well localized. S1 supplies the sole and the outer border of the leg and foot. L5 supplies the dorsum of the foot and the anterior aspect of the lower leg, and L4 the anteromedial aspect of the thigh (fig. 8.7). The correct evaluation of sensory appreciation demands, strangely enough, a meticulous technique. Only gross changes can be detected by the perfunctory jab of a pin. When minor changes are sought it is important to remember that sensory appreciation is dependent on summation of stimuli. Because of this physiological phenomenon, 10 pinpricks applied to a partially denervated area of the skin may be appreciated as readily as one or two pinpricks on the opposite leg. For accurate evaluation, the "stimulus" applied should be the same in both areas under comparison.

Vibration sensibility below the knees is not as acute over the age of 50 and the same applies to temperature appreciation. It must be remembered that the demonstration of a stocking type of diminished appreciation of pinprick does not necessarily indicate that the pain is hysterical in origin. It may merely indicate that the patient is demonstrating a hysterical exaggeration of signs derived from a significant organic lesion. The significance of such a demonstration of sensory loss must be evaluated with all other symptoms and signs presented by the patient.

Signs of root tension may now be evaluated. Root tension is a term reserved to denote reproduction of pain by stretching a peripheral nerve. When testing the sciatic nerve the leg must never be raised suddenly by lifting the heel, because so much pain may be evoked by this maneuver as to make all other examinations useless. The leg should be raised slowly with the knee maintained in the fully extended position by the examiner's hands (fig. 8.8). It is important to record the range through which the leg must be raised before pain is experienced. Reproduction of pain in this manner does not necessarily indicate root tension, of course. With any painful lesion of the back associated with hamstring spasm, straight leg raising will rotate the pelvis and irritate the lumbosacral region, giving rise to pain. However, reproduction or aggravation of sciatic pain by forced dorsiflexion of the ankle at the limit of straight leg raising is highly suggestive of root tension, and this impression is confirmed if the patient admits relief on bending the knee. If a patient still has pain after the knee has been flexed and if the pain is increased on further flexion of the

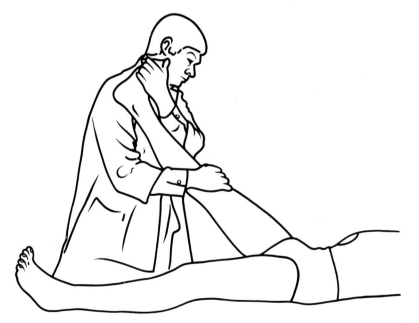

Fig. 8.8. When carrying out the straight leg raising test, it is important to remember that the leg should be raised *slowly* and during this movement, the knee must be maintained in the fully extended position by the examiner's hand.

hip (bent leg raising), then the examiner should be concerned that he is dealing with a patient suffering from a significant emotional breakdown or else there may be a lesion of the hip joint presenting as sciatic pain.

Straight leg raising of the opposite leg, the symptom-free leg, giving rise to an exacerbation of pain in the affected extremity, is very suggestive of a massive disc herniation, usually lying medial to the root.

The most reliable test of root tension is the bowstring sign. In this test, straight leg raising is carried out until pain is reproduced. At this level, the knee is slightly flexed until the pain abates. The examiner rests the limb on his shoulder and places his thumbs in the popliteal fossa over the sciatic nerve. If sudden firm pressure on the nerve gives rise to pain in the back or down the leg, the patient is almost certainly suffering from significant root tension (fig. 8.9).

In a patient with weak abdominal muscles and disc degeneration, attempts to perform bilateral active straight leg raising are painful because the weight of the legs rotates the pelvis causing hyperextension of the lumbar spine (fig. 8.10).

Flexion of the hip with the knee flexed should not aggravate a mechanical back pain, but patients with emotional breakdowns frequently complain bitterly during this maneuver.

At this stage of the examination the full range of hip joint movements

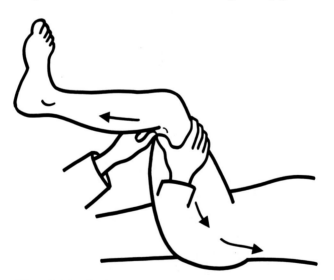

Fig. 8.9. When eliciting the Bowstring sign the patient's foot should be allowed to rest on the examiner's shoulder with the knee very slightly flexed at the limit of straight leg raising. Sudden firm pressure is then applied by the examiner's thumbs in the popliteal fossa. Radiation of pain down the leg or the production of pain in the back is pathognomonic of root tension.

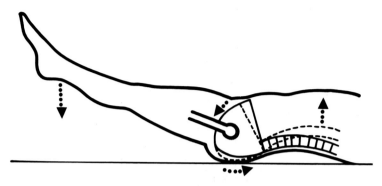

Fig. 8.10. When the patient carries out bilateral active straight leg raising, the weight of the legs causes the pelvis to rotate and thereby hyperextends the lumbar spine. Hyperextension of the lumbar spine in the presence of disc degeneration gives rise to pain. This is probably the most useful test to demonstrate the presence of painful segmental instability.

should be assessed. Osteoarthritis of the hip joint may give rise to symptoms and signs mimicking fourth lumbar root compression: pain down the front of the thigh, weakness and atrophy of the quadriceps, tenderness on palpation of the quadriceps, pain on the femoral nerve stretch test. This confusion arises from perfunctory examination. *Always* assess hip joint motion fully.

With the patient still supine, the abdomen is palpated for evidence of intra-abdominal masses and the peripheral pulses are palpated for evidence of vascular insufficiency.

The patient is then turned on his side. The ability to abduct the leg against resistance is tested. When this movement is performed, the glutei must contract vigorously and tend to pull the pelvis away from the sacrum. A patient with a sacroiliac strain or any sacroiliac disease will find this movement painful.

The sacroiliac joint can also be tested by applying a rotary strain. The unaffected hip joint is flexed and the thigh held firmly against the chest by the patient in order to lock the lumbar spine. The uppermost hip is now extended to its limit. When pushed beyond the limit of hip joint extension, a rotary strain is applied to the sacroiliac joint, a movement that causes pain with sacroiliac diseases (fig. 8.11). Sometimes in a sacroiliac joint lesion, lateral compression of the pelvis with the patient lying on his side gives rise to pain.

It is frequently convenient, because the patient is already on his side, to carry out a rectal examination at this stage.

The patient is turned face downward and the buttocks and thighs are palpated for tumors involving the sciatic nerve.

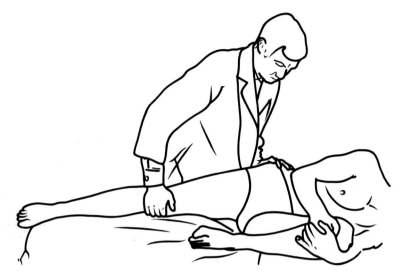

Fig. 8.11. Gaenslen's test. The patient lies on his side and holds his lumbar spine rigid by flexing his lowermost hip and pulling his knee against his chest. The uppermost hip is now extended by the examiner. At the limit of hip joint extension, any further extension strain applies a rotary strain to the pelvis and tends to rotate one-half of the ilium against the sacrum. With sacroiliac joint lesions, this maneuver is painful.

This test can also be performed with the patient lying on his back holding his knee flexed against his chest and a hyperextension strain can be applied to the hip by allowing the leg to drop over the side of the table.

In lesions involving the third and fourth lumbar roots, the patient will experience pain on stretching the femoral nerve. This test can be performed with the patient lying face downward. The hip is then extended, with the knee maintained in a slightly flexed position. This test is only of significance if the patient experiences pain radiating down the front of the thigh (fig. 8.12).

Care must be taken not to confuse the femoral nerve stretch test with Ely's sign. Ely's sign was designed to demonstrate contracture or shortening of the rectus femoris. The rectus femoris spans both the hip joint and the knee joint, flexing the hip and extending the knee. When the knee is fully flexed, the rectus femoris is stretched. If there is any contracture of the muscle, passive stretching in this manner will cause the hip to flex. This can be easily demonstrated by fully flexing the knee with the patient lying face downward, when the resulting flexion of the hip is shown by the fact that the buttock rises off the bed. This is Ely's test. This test is frequently positive in patients of mesomorphic build. In some patients suffering from fourth lumbar root irritation, this maneuver gives rise to severe quadriceps pain.

At this stage of the examination, a tape measure is used. Leg lengths are measured. The maximal girth of the calf is compared on the two sides and the circumference of the thigh measured on both sides at a fixed distance from the tibial tubercle. The patient is then asked to sit on the side of the couch so that chest expansion can be determined. A decrease in chest expansion is an early change in ankylosing spondylitis.

The patient is now asked to step down from the couch and drape himself over its edge, resting the abdomen on a pillow. This position is usually comfortable and brings all the spinous processes into prominence. An area not expected to be tender is tested first. Firm pressure applied to the spine may be uncomfortable. The patient must be able to differentiate between the expected discomfort of such pressure and the abnormal discomfort when the damaged segment is palpated. Each spinous process is palpated separately with firm pressure being exerted anteriorly *and in a lateral direction* (fig. 8.13).

Although the specific findings on examination of patients suffering from psychogenic regional pain are discussed in detail in chapter 11, physical signs of emotional overtones are so commonly overlooked they cannot be overemphasized and are separately tabulated at this point. The following points noted on examination should make the clinician wary of the possibility of significant emotional overtones:

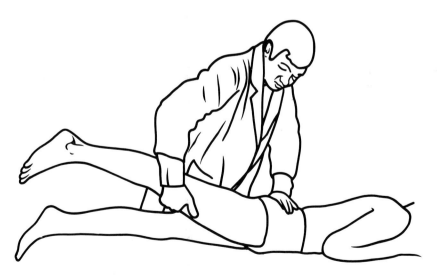

Fig. 8.12. When the fourth lumbar nerve root is compromised, the patient experiences pain radiating down the front of the thigh. This pain will be aggravated if the hip is extended with the knees slightly flexed. It is to be noted that this test may give rise to back pain by virtue of hyperextending the spine, but this finding is not of diagnostic significance.

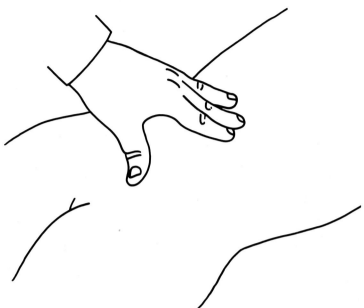

Fig. 8.13. Pain on direct pressure over a spinous process may reflect nothing more than referred tenderness. More information can be obtained if the examiner places his thumb against the side of the spinous process and applies pressure not only in a forward direction but in a lateral direction as well, thereby applying a rotary strain to the segment. Reproduction of the clinically experienced pain by this maneuver is of great diagnostic significance.

1. Walking painfully slowly, leaning heavily on a cane.
2. The insistence of having his wife (or her husband) corroborate the history.
3. Pathetic slowness in movement, walking unsurely as though in a darkened room.
4. "Play acting": a dramatic display of distress when pain is elicited. Very few people "hurt that badly."
5. When movements of the spine are being examined, the patient may bend forward or backward very, very slowly and suddenly and unexpectedly give a violent jerk to denote the experience of pain. Such a jerk would normally aggravate the pain immensely and is in reality a further example of the histrionic or play-acting response.
6. Inability to increase the range of flexion of the lumbar spine even when kneeling on a chair. When the patient is kneeling, the hamstrings and sciatic nerves are relaxed and the patient should be able to bend forward with a fair degree of comfort

even in the presence of marked root tension. The only exceptions to this rule, of course, are patients suffering from vertebral
osteomyelitis or from ankylosing spondylitis.

7. Pain on straight leg raising not relieved by flexion of the knee
   and aggravated by further flexion of the hip with the knee flexed.
   The examiner, of course, must be careful that he is not missing
   an osteoarthritis of the hip joint.
8. "Cogwheel" weakness of muscle groups. The "give-away"
   weakness that is a give-away of an emotional response.
9. Tenderness on pinching the skin. This tenderness is generally
   most marked over the major area of pain.
10. Hypoesthesia to pinprick over nonanatomical distributions.
    The stocking anesthesia is generally readily recognized. The
    physician may omit sensory examination on the area of the
    maximal pain in the back. The demonstration of a square of
    hypoesthesia in relation to the site of back pain is highly sug-
    gestive of emotional overtones.

RADIOLOGICAL EXAMINATION

The question always arises, "Should an x-ray be taken?" An x-ray is
not harmful, but it is about as illogical to take an x-ray of every patient
who has a backache as it is to order a barium meal on everyone who has a
touch of indigestion. An x-ray on the first attendance of a patient with
back pain is, however, indicated under the following circumstances:

1. Severe back pain following significant trauma.
2. Incapacitating back pain.
3. A history suggestive of vertebral crush due to osteoporosis or
   malignancy. These patients, usually over the age of 50, give a
   history of pain coming on without provocative injury, punctuated
   by sudden cramps of pain in the back.
4. The excessively anxious patient. In such people the taking of an
   x-ray is an essential part of treatment. They cannot be reassured
   by clinical examination alone.
5. Patients in whom the history and examination are suggestive of
   ankylosing spondylitis. A specific request should be made for
   oblique views of the sacroiliac joint.
6. Patients with a clinically apparent spinal deformity.
7. Patients with significant root tension and patients presenting
   evidence of impairment of root conduction. In these patients, an
   x-ray is of importance to exclude the possibility of malignancy.
8. If severe pain persists despite treatment for more than 2 weeks,
   then an x-ray is indicated, not only to exclude the possibility of

some obscure spinal abnormality but also to reassure the patient that he is not suffering from a serious progressive disease.

X-rays have a limited function in diagnosis and treatment. In diagnosis, the main function of an x-ray is to exclude serious disease, such as infections, ankylosing spondylitis, and neoplasms. If x-rays of the spine show disc degeneration, this radiological change merely demonstrates a segment that is vulnerable to trauma. Such a demonstration, however, does not necessarily indict this segment as the cause of the presenting symptoms. Treatment is determined by clinical assessment, not by the radiological findings.

Radiological examination of the spine carries with it certain dangers. Anatomical anomalies demonstrated on x-ray may stop any further thought on the part of the physician. These anomalies are rarely the cause of back pain but are a frequent cause of anxiety in patients told of their presence. Even the statement "your x-rays showed degenerative discs" may induce unpleasant misapprehension in the patient.

The term "degeneration" implies to the average patient a type of "rotting away," like bad cheese. A patient should never be presented with the bald statement "the x-rays of your spine show arthritis." First, this is rarely true. The presence of osteophytes or, more correctly, "spondylophytes" on the vertebral bodies does not denote arthritis. Second, the term "arthritis" carries with it an evil connotation for the patient. Given this diagnosis, the patients frequently foresee a progressive restriction in their way of life leading eventually to a wheelchair existence.

Detailed assessment of radiological findings indicative of mechanical insufficiency of the spine is only of value in the preoperative assessment of a patient. At this time, a thorough analysis of the x-ray findings is of importance in determining whether surgical intervention is feasible and in determining the type of operative correction required.

CHAPTER 9

Disc Degeneration without Root Irritation

"It is easy to get a thousand prescriptions but hard to get a single remedy."

—Anonymous

Before any treatment is started, we must know why the patient seeks advice, why the patient is so disabled by the pain, and what goal can be set for treatment.

Let us consider the first important question, "Why has this patient come to seek advice?" Many patients have seen relatives in the terminal phases of malignancy whose last major symptom was backache. Others have friends or relatives with rheumatoid arthritis. The development of pain in the back without provocative incident may be a frightening experience for these people. The pain may be perfectly tolerable, little more than nuisance value. They do not require, nor are they asking for, specific treatment. They need, and need badly, a diagnosis. They need to know the cause of their worrisome complaint.

With reassurance that they do not have cancer, with reassurance that they do not have arthritis, many are perfectly content to carry on with normal activities with the knowledge that in the course of time, without specific therapy, their symptoms will subside.

The second important question to answer is "Why is this patient so disabled by the pain that he is describing?" Emotional overlays are very common, and it is important for the physician to try and assess whether he is dealing with an emotionally labile patient who has developed back pain; whether the back pain, by virtue of interfering with the patient's ability to get on with his normal way of life and by virtue of interfering with his capacity to earn an income, has produced secondary emotional features; or whether, indeed, the patient's somatic complaints are just one facet of a general emotional breakdown.

The question of the significance of emotional factors is always brought to the forefront when it appears to the clinician, on taking the history and on examining the patient, that the disability complained of is out of proportion to the possible pathological changes that could have taken place.

Finally, it is always necessary to set a goal in treatment. Physicians set goals for the total management of patients with coronary thrombosis: they do not return to professional football. Physicians set goals for patients with hypertension or even increasing nerve deafness. We must also recognize our limitations in the management of degenerative disease of the lumbar spine, and we must be prepared to set realistic goals.

The goal in a young man with his first acute episode of sciatica is to return him to normal activities. The goal with an overweight, overwrought, unskilled laborer who has not yet learned the language of the country of adoption may be merely to add to the painless unemployed.

Every patient will present with his own personal peculiar problems: "I'm getting married this afternoon, Doctor." Although treatment must, of course, be individualized, certain guidelines may be laid down. These guidelines do not have a firm scientific foundation: they are based on experience empirically acquired. They represent, therefore, a philosophy of management rather than a dogma of treatment and, as such, must be constantly modified by the special needs of the society in which you work and by your increasing experience with the special problems that these people face.

For discussion of the treatment of discogenic back pain, it is best to consider the clinical manifestations of disc degeneration under two headings: disc degeneration without root irritation and disc degeneration associated with root irritation.

The clinical syndromes resulting from disc degeneration may be considered under five specific headings: acute incapacitating, recurrent aggravating, chronic persisting, psychogenic magnification, and cervicolumbar syndrome.

ACUTE INCAPACITATING BACKACHE

There are not many people who have lived for a half century who have not, at some time in their lives, been smitten by an acute episode of incapacitating backache. Perversely this is encouraging. These people do not remain incapacitated: they get better, perhaps despite treatment rather than because of it.

Characteristically, the patient while engaged in some trivial activity is suddenly seized with back pain and cannot move. "I was paralyzed with pain." The lumbar spine is splinted rigidly and the patient can only move with painful caution, clutching his back and walking with his trunk leaning forward, keeping his hips and knees slightly bent.

Examination reveals that all movements of the spine are limited by pain and muscle spasm, but there is no evidence of root tension.

The clinical picture is explosively dramatic and threatening to the patient. The physician must not over-react. The physician must constantly remind himself that even if he elected to treat the patient by rubbing peanut butter on each buttock, in the balance of probabilities, the patient would get well, fairly quickly.

In the majority of such cases the patient is suffering from a "sprain" of one of the zygapophysial joints. When trying to rationalize treatment, one should compare the lesion with a severely sprained ankle in a patient who has only one leg and who is unable to wear a prosthesis. There is only one way to treat a sprained ankle in such a patient: the patient has to be put to bed. Theoretically, the patient with an acute low back strain should also be treated by strict bedrest. However, theoretical treatment must be tempered by reason. If your patient is a young housewife, who is going to look after the children? Who is going to get the meals? What about tomorrow's office for the dentist with an acute back pain?

Let me repeat once again: you are treating a patient and not a spine and the experience of the lay world is that many, in fact, the majority, will get better by just creeping around, with their pain mollified by analgesics.

Some patients, however, can't cope. The pain is too severe. In such instances, if they can't do their normal daily work they should be sent to bed.

A patient with pneumonia is ill and defeated: he is happy to go to bed. A patient with a severe low back pain feels well in himself and doesn't want to go to bed. He is hopping mad at his affliction and your insistence on bedrest will increase his frustration, unless you take care and take time to explain in detail the purpose of this apparently neglectful form of management. It is advisable to give him some literature explaining in detail the probable underlying pathology and the rationale of treatment by bedrest (table 9.1). You must advise the patient in regard to toilet facilities. Using a bedpan at home is impractical. The use of crutches makes it easier for the patient to get to the bathroom and the purchase of a high toilet seat is sometimes essential.

Although analgesics are rarely needed once the patient is in bed, in the majority, sedatives (tranquilizers, if you will) are essential. At present there is no specific medication to speed the resolution of the symptoms, although anti-inflammatory drugs may help some patients.

The question of the role of manipulation is always raised. The "locking" of the back by spasm of the paraspinal muscles may tend to perpetuate the problem and gentle flexion of the spine into the fetal

Table 9.1. Instructions for Patients on the Purpose of Bedrest

---

Many patients with an acute incapacitating back pain are surprised when they are told that the only significant form of treatment is complete bedrest. This does not appear to be treatment at all. It almost seems like neglectful indifference on the part of the physician.

Your must remember that the spine is a column made of blocks of bone connected together by small joints and that an acute mechanical backache is in reality simply a severely sprained joint. It gives rise to pain in the same way that a severe sprain of the ankle gives rise to pain. With a sprained ankle, however, you can limp and continue to get around by taking the weight off the injured joint, while putting most of your weight on the other leg.

However, if a patient with only one leg sprains his ankle, he can't limp. He can't take the weight off his injured foot. He can't walk around. He has to go to bed until the "inflammation" of the sprain settles down.

The same applies to the spine. You have only one spine, and when you severely sprain the joints in your spine, the only way to take the weight and strain of activities away from the spinal joints is to lie down.

Therefore, bedrest is rational treatment. It is the quickest way to recovery.

---

position of rest appears to release the muscle hyperactivity. This is best accomplished initially by getting the patient to flex his knees and hips and then use his hands to pull the knees against the chest repetitively (fig. 9.1). Later, a passive flexion manipulation can be carried out. The patient lies on his back with his hips and knees flexed. His heels are grasped so that his feet point toward the ceiling. The feet are then pushed gently over the patient's head. This movement is repeated slowly and rhythmically. This repetitive rocking must be carried out with slow simple harmonic motion with each swing of the legs flexing the spine a little further. This rhythmical swinging is continued for about 2 minutes (fig. 9.2).

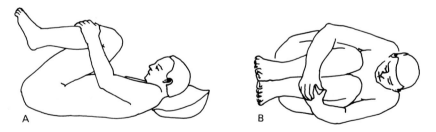

Fig. 9.1. A patient may abort an acute episode of low back pain by lying on his back and pulling his knees slowly up to his chest (*A*). He should maintain this position for 5 minutes. In very acute attacks with severe pain the patient may find it easier to assume the same position lying on his side (*B*).

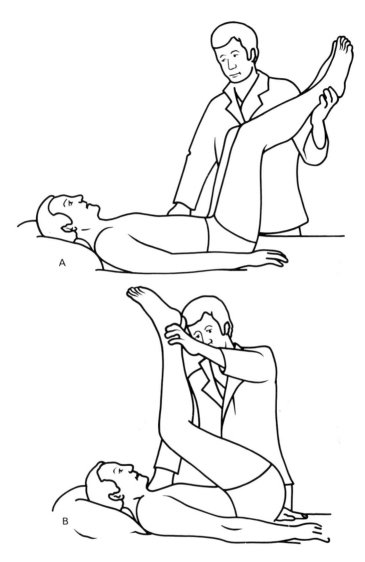

Fig. 9.2. If, on clinical examination, there is no evidence of root compression, resolution of symptoms may be speeded by a flexion manipulation. The patient lies on his back and the physician raises the patient's legs maintaining the knees in flexion (A). By applying pressure to the heels the physician then pushes the patient's knees towards the shoulders (B). This movement is done very slowly and the degree of flexion obtained is determined by the discomfort the patient experiences. This movement is then repeated slowly and rhythmically over a period of 5 minutes. In the majority of instances, the range of movement that can be achieved by this passive manipulation gradually increases. At the conclusion of the manipulation, the patient is instructed to flex his knees fully and allow his feet to come down to the bed, soles first.

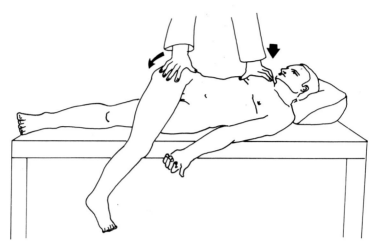

Fig. 9.3. Rotation manipulation.

This is a much more effective maneuver for the occasional manipulator than the specific manipulation of spinous processes or the commonly employed flexion rotation manipulation of the lumbosacral joint (fig. 9.3).

To be effective, however, this manipulative therapy must continue on a daily basis and, therefore, the patient must learn how to perform these maneuvers by himself. The patient should be taught specific steps. The manipulation exercises are carried out on a bed, not on the floor. The neck is kept slightly flexed by a pillow to minimize the effects of the inevitable contraction of the sternomastoids when the patients first make their attempts to kick their feet up in the air.

The hips and knees are first flexed to a right angle. The legs are then raised toward the ceiling, keeping the knees slightly bent. The patient then attempts to move his feet over his head. This movement must not be in the form of a sudden kick. The buttocks must be raised slowly and smoothly off the bed by contraction of the trunk flexors and then, just as slowly, the legs are lowered. This movement is repeated several times, each time lowering legs just to the starting position with the hips flexed at 90°. *The legs must not be lowered to the bed.*

After five "kick-ups," the patient rests by lowering his legs, with the knees fully flexed, thereby putting his feet onto the bed, soles first (fig. 9.4).

This routine, at this stage in the treatment of an acute back pain, is not designed to be an exercise program. It is really an active flexion manipulation of the spine. The duration of these flexion manipulations should be restricted to 10 kick-ups only and these should be repeated three times a day.

Bedrest should be continued until the patient can make his journeys to the toilet in relative comfort without the aid of crutches. After this period of time, the patient gradually increases his activities within the limits set by his own tolerance of decreasing discomforts. The time of return to work is determined largely by the demands made on the patient's back by his job.

Some time ago there was a vogue for the use of plaster body jackets in the treatment of the acute incapacitating discogenic backache. However, if the patient cannot work wearing a body jacket, he's better off lying in bed. Plaster jackets may still have a place in the treatment of patients in whom it is virtually impossible to take any time off work. It is the second

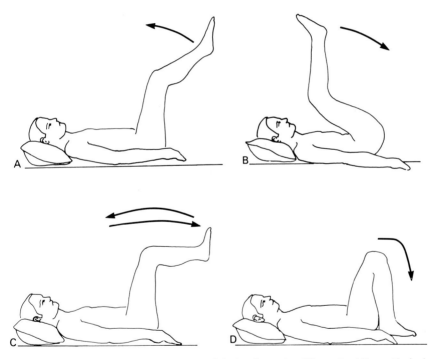

Fig. 9.4. Flexion exercise-manipulation of the lumbar spine. The patient lies on the bed with the head supported by a pillow. The hips are flexed to 90° and the knees slightly flexed (A). The patient now attempts to kick the feet over the head, raising the buttocks approximately 6 inches off the bed (B). After each "kick-up" the patient returns to the starting position (C). After five kick-ups, the patient rests by lowering his legs with the knees fully flexed, thereby putting his feet on the bed, soles first (D). It is very important that he should not lower the legs with the knees fully extended because this places a painful hyperextension strain on the spine.

best form of treatment and, to be of any value at all, very rigid criteria must be met. The most important of these is that the patient must be able to work and to travel to and from work while wearing the jacket.

The jacket must be applied very snugly with pressure points well protected.

While the jacket is being applied, an attempt must be made to flatten the lumbar spine. This can be achieved by having the patient stand with one foot on a stool. The plaster must be molded so it presses into the abdomen, and by increasing abdominal pressure, unweights the spine (fig. 9.5).

The jacket must be contoured so it fits snugly over the lower rib margin and over the iliac crest to prevent it from sliding up and down when the patient changes position.

It is not an easy plaster to apply and, indeed, it is a desperation measure designed solely to meet a specific demand, the need to stay at light work despite apparently incapacitating backache. There is no point in keeping the plaster jacket on for more than 1 week or 10 days. If the patient is still grossly incapacitated at the end of this time, the jacket should be removed and the patient should be sent to bed. If the gods have

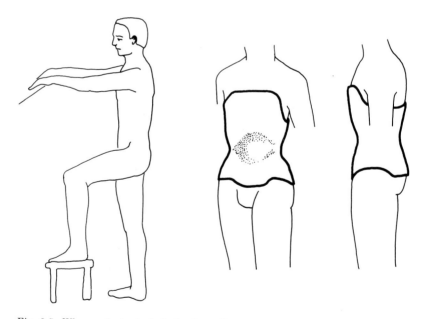

Fig. 9.5. When a plaster body jacket is applied for the treatment of low back pain, the lumbar spine should be flattened by making the patient stand with one foot on a stool. The front of the cast should press firmly against the abdomen to increase intra-abdominal pressure and thereby "unweight" the spine.

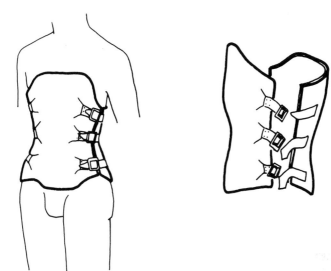

Fig. 9.6. The use of webbing straps and buckles allows the patient to remove and reapply a plaster body jacket during the acute phase of low back pain.

smiled at your Olympian efforts and the pain has abated somewhat, then the plaster should be bivalved and over the next 3 weeks worn during the day, while at work, being held in position by webbing straps (fig. 9.6).

When the smoke of the battle has cleared away and the patient is now relatively pain-free, he will always ask, "What is there to prevent me from getting another attack like this one?" This is a very reasonable question. Fortunately, severe recurrences are not nearly as common as might be anticipated. Many just have one attack. Predisposing factors must be checked. Weight is a major offender and you must not let your patients eat their way into the restrictive life of spinal rule.

Adequate trunk muscles are the major guardians against repeated attacks. It must be remembered that the spinal column is not a self-supporting structure. If the trunk and abdominal muscles are paralyzed, such as in infantile paralysis, the spine collapses. The spine is supported by muscle action in much the same way that the mast of a ship is supported by stays (fig. 9.7). In addition to this, the abdominal cavity acts as a hydraulic sac, dissipating loads by pressing upward on the diaphragm and downward on the pelvic floor, thereby unweighting the spine (fig. 9.8). Because of this, the tone and strength of the abdominal muscles are of vital importance in protecting the spine against weight-bearing and extension strains.

Patients who have had back pain severe enough to warrant 2 weeks in

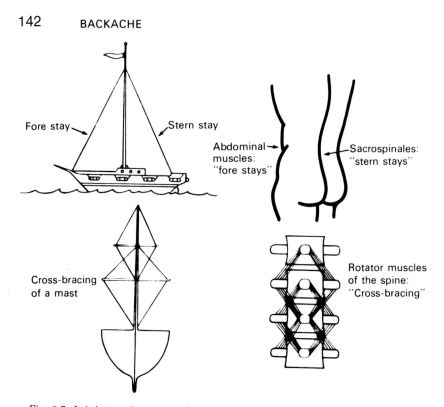

Fig. 9.7. It is interesting to note the similarity between the bracing used to support the mast of a ship and the muscular bracing of the human spine.

bed and marked modification of their daily activities for a further month should continue the flexion manipulation exercises, previously described, for 1 year. The patients must aim at carrying out 50 kick-ups once a day and this program must be rigidly adhered to, with almost religious fervor.

There are many other exercise programs, of course, but time is of importance. If the physical therapy program given to the patient is too ambitious, if it takes 1/2 to 1 hour or more to complete, the patient will rarely continue to carry it out. It is better that they should be started on a program that they will be willing to continue on a daily basis for a year rather than a more vigorous program that they will get fed up with in about 1 month.

The essence of permanent cure is to try to persuade the patients to increase their generally physical activities. Some patients claim, and probably rightly so, that their nagging backache prevents them from doing this and some of these people may be helped by the provision of a brace. I have stated "*some* of these people" advisedly. A brace is not a panacea that helps all discogenic backache and, therefore, before ordering one, consider the mode of action of any spinal support.

A brace will not hold up a spine; most are not strong enough to hold up a rose bush. The most important component of a spinal brace is the abdominal binder (fig. 9.9). In the obese patient, the center of gravity is a long way in front of the vertebral column, and the lumbar spine must be hyperextended in order that the patient can stand erect. A tight corset, by pushing the center of gravity nearer the spine, enables the patient to decrease the lordotic curve. However, if, as is frequently the case in the commonly employed braces, the rigid posterior steels are bent in to fit the lordotic curve, then this important function is lost and, indeed, the pressure of the steel supports against the back may increase the discomfort.

I have grave doubts as to the value of the rigid steel supports. They do not significantly restrict movement. They do not unweight the spine, and the main function of the vertical supports is merely to prevent the garment from wrinkling. This function can be equally subserved by flexible steels which at the same time will allow compression of the abdomen and flattening of the lumbar spine.

Compression of the abdomen has the important function of increasing intra-abdominal pressure, thereby pushing up on the diaphragm and down on the pelvic floor and by so doing unweighting the spine. It is of interest to note that by giving firm pressure on the skin, any tight garment makes the patients feel better; this is probably due to type A nerve fiber stimulation. This is a common experience. When you hit your

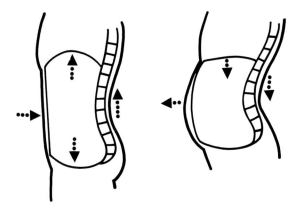

Fig. 9.8. The abdominal cavity acts in a manner similar to a hydraulic sac. By increasing intra-abdominal pressure, the diaphragm is pushed up and the pelvic floor is pushed down. This tends to "elongate" the lumbar spine, thereby taking some of the weight off the discs and the posterior joints.

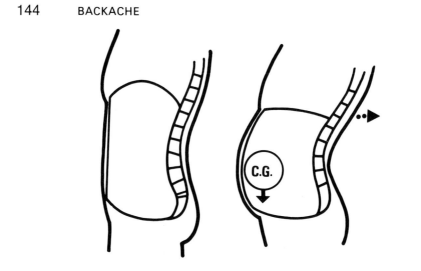

Fig. 9.9. Obesity, by pulling the center of gravity forward, causes the spine to hyperextend.

thumb with a hammer you squeeze it. When you have a headache you press on the side of the temples. Patients with a backache squeeze their loins with their hands and feel better. This is part of the action of a corset.

A useful corset then must have a strong anterior binder capable of applying firm pressure to the abdomen. Although corset design is of importance, the shape of the patient is of equal importance. If the patient is very thin, if she has high iliac crests and a narrow waist and a prominent flared-out lower rib margin, it is impossible with corsets presently available to apply significant abdominal pressure. A corset in such a patient would expend its compressive effect on the ribs or on the pelvis and, therefore, fail to give relief. The overweight and chubby patients achieve the greatest benefit from the provision of a corset.

The function of the corset must be explained to the patient. It is useless just to sling it around the waist like a talisman; it must be worn very tightly and the patient must be instructed that he must gradually get himself accustomed to the high abdominal pressure that is required.

RECURRENT AGGRAVATING BACKACHE

This is probably the most common manifestation of disc degeneration associated with segmental instability or segmental hyperextension. Rowe, studying the incidence of low back pain in workers at the Kodak Company, found that 85% of the patients with backache had intermittent attacks of disabling pain every 3 months to 3 years, each attack lasting 3 days to 3 weeks. Between the attacks, the patients were relatively free from backache. Most of these patients were suffering from recurrent hyperextension strains of a posterior joint. The posterior joints are vulnerable to extension strains because degenerative changes in one or more discs may give rise to segmental hyperextension or persistent posterior joint subluxation. The facets of the involved segment or segments in these conditions are held at the extreme limit of extension; they have no safety factor of movement. A simple analogy can be drawn with the wrist. If a moderate blow is applied to the palm of the hand with the wrist in the neutral position, no pain results because the force of the blow is absorbed by the movement that occurs. If, however, the hand is hit with the same force, with the wrist in full extension, then this is painful because there is no safety factor of movement and the full brunt of the injury is transmitted to the capsule of the wrist (fig. 9.10).

The same mechanical principle applies to the spine. In the neutral position moderate extension strains are not painful, but if a segment is held in hyperextension there is no safety factor in movement and the extension strains of everyday living give rise to painful capsular lesions.

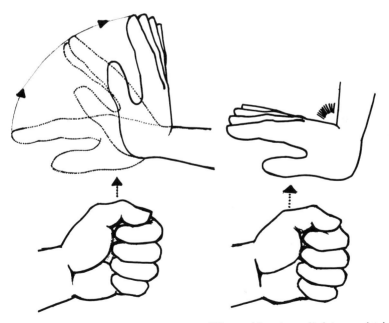

Fig. 9.10. The safety factor of movement. When a blow is applied to a wrist in the neutral position, the force of the blow is absorbed by the movement that occurs. When the same force is applied to the wrist in dorsiflexion, pain results because there is no safety factor of movement and the full force of the blow is felt by the capsule of the wrist joint.

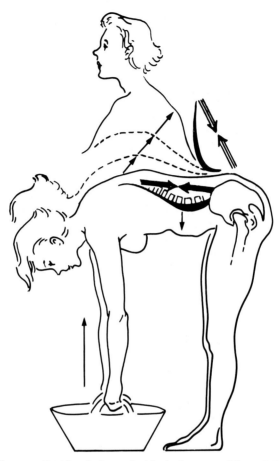

Fig. 9.11. When a patient bends forward with the knees straight and then tries to lift, the sacrospinales, when contracting, act as a bowstring and hyperextend the lumbar spine.

The significance of extension strains is noted both in the history and in the examination of the patient.

Working with the hands above the head, such as in hanging up laundry, reaching, etc., applies extension strains to the back and is painful. When the forward stooped position is maintained, the sacrospinales have to contract to hold the spine. With an unstable lumbar disc segment, in this position, the sacrospinales act as a bowstring producing hyperextension at the involved segment (fig. 9.11). These patients complain of pain on stooping over the washbasin in the morning and when maintaining the bent forward position, as when making beds, etc.

Sitting in a soft chair will allow the lumbar spine to concertina and sag into hyperlordosis. These patients find it more comfortable to sit on a hard seat. Sitting in a theater with the knees out straight and the floor sloping away will apply a significant extension strain to the spine and the patients tend to irritate the patrons in the row in front, by putting their feet on the back of their seat, in order to keep their knees and hips flexed. Similarly, sitting in a car with the knees held straight hyperextends the spine and prolonged driving is uncomfortable.

When these patients stand for long periods of time, the lumbar spine sags into extension and the patients automatically try to flatten the lumbar spine by flexing one hip and knee, as in the act of putting one foot on the seat of a chair or on a bar rail. Emotional tensions and frustrations will make the patient adopt the fight position, tightening up the sacrospinales. This posture will aggravate the pain, and the patient's increase in pain will aggravate his frustrations.

The pain experienced is commonly localized to the lumbosacral junction radiating out to one or both sacroiliac joints. If the pain intensifies it may radiate down one or both legs in a sciatic distribution as far as the knee. On occasion the pain may be experienced just over one sacroiliac joint or in one buttock. Occasionally the pain may radiate into the groin and, indeed, severe groin pain may be the major presenting symptom.

On examination the patients may demonstrate an increase in the normal lumbar lordosis, but more commonly they do not demonstrate any postural spinal abnormalities.

They may, however, show many mechanical features that tend to aggravate hyperextension of the lumbar spine.

Weak Abdominal Muscles

These patients have difficulty in doing sit-ups with their hips and knees bent and the palms of the hands clasped behind their heads. Because of the weakness of the abdominal muscles, when they lift both legs off the couch (bilateral straight leg raising), the weight of the legs tends to rotate the pelvis, hyperextending the spine and producing pain in the back (fig. 8.10). Back pain reproduced by bilateral active straight leg raising is probably the best demonstration of symptomatic lumbar disc degeneration aggravated by weak abdominal muscles.

Obesity

Excessive weight loading hyperextends the lumbar spine. This is particularly apparent in the patient who has an "alderman's pouch" (a protuberant fat abdomen). With the center of gravity anterior to the spine, the patient has to hyperextend his back to stand erect.

Tensor Fascia Femoris Contracture

Some patients, especially those with a mesomorphic build, have a tight tensor fascia femoris which tilts the pelvis forward (fig. 9.12). With the pelvis fixed in this position, the lumbar spine must hyperextend to allow the spinal column to remain erect. When these patients stand against the wall with the back of the head, chest, buttocks, and heels touching the wall, they cannot flatten their lumbar spine. The only way they can flatten their backs against a wall is to step forward and bend their knees, thereby relaxing the tensor fascia femoris and allowing the pelvis to rotate. On examination, adduction of the hip is markedly limited when the hip is internally rotated and extended at the same time.

Special note, then, is made of these aggravating factors: abdominal weakness, weight, and tightness of the tensor fascia femoris.

The physical findings in chronic degenerative disc disease are not very dramatic. If the patient is seen after the acute attack has subsided, movements of the lumbar spine may not be significantly limited. Forward flexion may be possible through a range that will allow the fingers to come within 18 inches of the floor. On extending from the forward flexed position, however, the patient generally shows reversal of normal spinal rhythm. After starting to extend their backs, they will bend their knees and hips to tuck their pelvis under the spine in order to regain the erect position (fig. 9.13). Extension in the erect position usually is limited and painful. If the examiner places his fingers on the anterior and posterior superior spines of the pelvis and then asks the

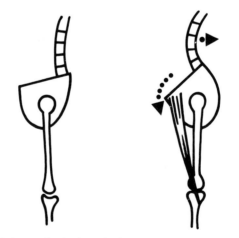

Fig. 9.12. A tight tensor fascia femoris, by rotating the pelvis anteriorly, produces hyperextension of the lumbar spine.

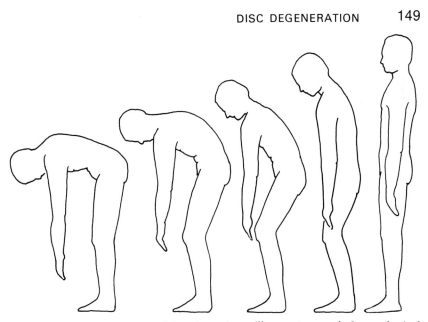

Fig. 9.13. With segmental instability the patient will present reversal of normal spinal rhythm on extending from the forward flexed position.

patient to bend backward, the pelvis can be felt to rotate after about 20° extension, and any further extension is painful.

Reversal of spinal rhythm on extending from the forward flexed position, pain on extension from the erect position, and pain on bilateral straight leg raising are common and, indeed, characteristic findings in chronic symptomatic degenerative disc disease. The demonstration of tenderness is not of significant diagnostic value and its distribution may be confusing. The injection of an irritating solution into the supraspinous ligament of L5 and S1 may give rise to local pain and also to pain referred to the sacroiliac joints and the buttocks or down the back of the thigh. Not only is pain referred in this distribution, but there may also be "referred tenderness." The upper outer quadrant of the buttock is normally tender on deep pressure. Following the injection of hypertonic saline into the supraspinous ligament between L5 and S1, the upper outer quadrant of buttock becomes extremely tender and this form of "central irritation" may produce tenderness over the sacroiliac joints and tenderness on pressure over the back of the thigh. The physician must not allow himself to be led to believe that the demonstration of a point of tenderness indicates that the pathology lies deep to this area. It was because of this common zone of tenderness over the sacroiliac joints associated with degenerative disc disease that the diagnosis of sacroiliac joint lesions became so popular about a half century ago.

In the treatment of recurrent aggravating discogenic back pain, the same general principles are employed as in the management of the acute incapacitating backache during its convalescent phase. Greater emphasis, of course, must be placed on the flexion exercise program, and on general physical training.

With recurrent episodes of back pain of an aggravating rather than incapacitating nature, a sense of frustration on the part of the physician may result in the patient being thrown into the garbage dump of undirected physical therapy. If you are going to employ the services of a physical therapist, you must do so with reason and purpose. Physical therapy should never be employed as a form of entertainment until such time as nature cures the symptoms. Heat in whatever modality employed, although making the patient feel better temporarily, does nothing to speed the resolution of the symptoms. To request massage is no more than using the physical therapy department as a medically approved body rub parlor.

Physical therapists can be sensibly and usefully employed to teach patients how to carry out an exercise program and to supervise their initial progress. Some patients are musculoskeletal morons. When trying to follow instructions on kick-up exercises, they look like a butterfly having an epileptic fit. These patients need help and direction; however, so do physical therapists. Never leave the exercise program to the discretion of the physical therapist. Rotation exercises may place undue stress on the discs and the posterior joints, and should only be undertaken by the very physically fit. Diverse corporal contortions may be inflicted on your patient which, although splendid in their place, should be kept in their place and reserved for the time when the patient has been symptom-free for many months.

Discuss the exercise program you want with your physical therapist, so that, for better or for worse, you will know what exercises your patients are doing. Some need instruction in muscular relaxation far more than they need instruction in muscular contraction. Probably one of the most useful roles of the physical therapist is to teach the patient the technique of voluntary muscular relaxation. Although you may send your patients to a physical therapy department, your aim is to get them out of the department as soon as possible. The time spent in journeying to the friendly physical therapist may constitute a greater disability than the discomfort itself. Put yourself in the patient's place. Do you want to take off what may be as long as 3 hours in your day, by the time you have driven to the physical therapy department, parked, waited for your turn, and then reversed the process? Try to get the patients to carry out the exercises at home.

The group of patients with a very tight tensor fascia femoris needs the help of a department of physical medicine. This postural defect has to be overcome by passive stretching of the muscle and for this you must have the help of a physical therapist.

CHRONIC PERSISTING BACKACHE

The *bete noire* of orthopedic surgeons is the syndrome of chronic, persisting discogenic low back pain, easily made intolerable by modest activity.

Patients with a chronic persistent daily backache generally give a history of having been plagued by intermittent episodes of back pain for several years. Eventually they reach the stage when the back pain never really leaves them. By driving themselves they may get through the average day with barely tolerable nagging discomfort in their back. They are very vulnerable to the traumatic insults of everyday life and, on minimal provocation, may get a "flare-up" of back pain. They have to be careful about everything they do and gradually, almost imperceptibly, their activities grind to a halt. They become the subjects of spinal rule, with their spine acting as a malevolent dictator determining what they can do and what they cannot do. These patients then give the history of a back pain that seriously interferes with their ability to do their work and their capacity to enjoy themselves in their leisure hours.

When assessing such patients it must be remembered that, although a chronic back pain may make the patient's life very miserable, persisting incapacitating back pain is most unusual. This first question that the physician has to ask himself then is "Why is *this* patient so disabled by the back pain she experiences?" It must be remembered that pain and disability are not synonymous. "The pain in my back is so severe I can't stoop to make the beds." This seems to be a perfectly reasonable complaint, but, nevertheless, it must be remembered that the patient is not describing the pain: she is describing her own reaction to the pain. Her next door neighbor with the same degree of pain may be out playing tennis. In chronic depressive states when the patient's emotional state is affected, the patient may describe an obviously unreasonable decrease of activities, "For the last 2 years the pain has been so bad that I have to use two canes to get around the house, and I haven't slept for more than 1 or 2 hours any night." This grossly exaggerated degree of disability is obviously divorced from reality. Discogenic back pain never gives rise to this degree of physical impairment for this length of time.

The magnification of the disability may be less bizarre. "I spend at least half the day lying down." "I can't walk a block." "I got a sudden severe attack of pain in the middle of the symphony concert and they had to carry me out on a stretcher."

Emotional problems commonly play a significant role in the disability resulting from chronic persistent low back pain. A patient with a hysterical personality tends to react hysterically to any pain, including a backache, but the histrionics generally subside as the pain abates. When the disability represents just one small facet of a general emotional breakdown, the symptoms will be intensified and perpetuated if too much attention is paid to them and too little attention is paid to the patient as a whole.

In the management of these patients then, the important questions to answer are: "Why is this patient so disabled by the pain he experiences?" "Where has the breakdown occurred—in the patient, or in the spine, or in both?"

Examination of the spine will reveal the features described in patients suffering from recurrent back pain due to segmental instability: pain on extension of the spine, reversal of normal spinal rhythm, pain on bilateral straight leg raising, and tenderness on palpation and manipulation of the lower lumbar spinous processes. It is frequently noted that the spinous processes do not separate very much on forward flexion.

Other factors contributing to the persistence of the pain may be noted: excessive weight, flabby abdominal muscles, a tight tensor fascia femoris. X-rays usually show the stigmata of degenerative disc disease at one or more segments.

No form of therapy will alter the degenerative changes that have occurred. Manipulation of the spine may result in a short-lived amelioration of symptoms, but rarely, if ever, gives rise to permanent relief.

In trying to outline a rational form of management of these patients, the following points must be remembered: (1) The natural tendency of the disease is toward recovery; (2) no specific treatment alters the changes in the disc; and (3) treatment perforce must be directed at making the patient comfortable while nature effects the cure.

When considering the means to make the patient comfortable, it must be remembered that (1) the pain is relieved by lying down, by unloading the spine; and (2) any activity that puts an extension strain on the spine increases the pain.

Bearing these two points in mind, patients can be managed by unloading the spine in the following manner:

1. Weight loss, where indicated.
2. Wearing a corset with a strong abdominal binder to increase intra-abdominal pressure and to bring the center of gravity nearer the spine.

3. Change of occupation. This course of action, although undesirable, may on occasion be the only realistic form of treatment. It most certainly must be considered in all heavy workers before considering a spinal fusion.

4. Teaching the patient to guard his spine against the extension strains of everyday living. The symptom of chronic persisting discogenic low back pain is almost invariably associated with fixed hyperextension of the zygapophysial joints resulting either from segmental hyperextension or from disc narrowing with posterior joint subluxation. The posterior joints are maintained at the limit of extension and any further attempt at extension is painful.

Extension strains are common: reaching, pushing, sitting with the legs out straight, prolonged standing, walking with big strides, etc. In the act of lifting with the knees straight, the sacrospinales act like a bowstring and extend the spine (fig. 9.11).

The patients must be taught to modify activities and assume postures that maintain the lumbar spine in the neutral position. They must be given written instructions in this regard (tables 9.2 and 9.3).

Extension strains are more liable to occur if the trunk flexors are weak, and a prolonged program to build up the trunk flexors is an essential part of treatment. The kick-up exercise-manipulation program is the simplest to learn and the one most readily accomplished and persevered with by the patient.

A corset should not be prescribed early in treatment. Flexion exercises and the flexion routine should be tried first and, as long as the patient shows some measure of improvement, they should be continued. If the patient reaches a plateau in recovery and is still plagued by back pain, then a corset should be ordered.

As mentioned previously, patients derive the most benefit from a corset with a strong abdominal binder worn tightly, but a simple canvas corset cannot produce significant compression of the abdomen in thin patients, especially if they have a prominent rib cage. The most that can be done for these patients is to try to restrict movement to some extent with a high thoracopelvic brace. The upper part of the brace must grasp the patient firmly around the lower rib cage and the pelvic band must fit snugly just below the iliac crest. Side and posterior steel supports will protect the patient, to some extent, against sudden jolts and jars. The posterior steel supports should not be curved in but should run in a straight line. The abdominal binder should be padded so that some pressure can be exerted against the abdominal wall (fig. 9.14).

Once the back pain is under some control, an increase in daily physical activities is an essential part of treatment. To be really effective, the progress of the patient must be checked regularly by the physician or by the physical therapist for a year. The treatment of a chronic, grumbling persistent back pain is like the treatment of a chronic alcoholic: nothing can be achieved during a single 15-minute consultation. If you are willing to follow these patients through, or get a team to do this, then in the well motivated patient the result will be worth the effort.

Table 9.2. Instructions for Male Patients on Flexion Routine

General Observations

Whenever possible, sit down. Sit with the knees higher than the hips. The best way of doing this is to sit with the feet on a footstool. If no footstool is available, then cross the legs. Never sit with the legs out straight.

Don't reach.

Dont't lift weights above the head.

Don't stoop.

Don't move furniture by pulling it in front of you.

Don't push windows up.

Don't put on weight.

Don't get overtired.

Don't maintain any one position for a prolonged period.

Sleeping

The mattress should be firm. If the mattress is soft, a board should be placed underneath it. Sleep on your side with your hips and knees bent.

Sitting

When driving a car the seat should be as close to the steering wheel as possible, thereby flexing the knees and hips. When riding in a car as a passenger, you should put a pillow behind your back so that you sit forward in the seat, again flexing the knees and hips. Whenever possible throughout the day, you should sit down with your knees higher than your hips in the "lazy boy" position.

Getting Up from Sitting

It is important not to arch the back on the act of getting up from sitting. Move to the front of the chair and stand up, keeping your back straight. Use your hands to help you if necessary.

Standing

The best way to stand is to adopt the posture commonly seen in a hotel: one foot on the ground and one foot on the brass rail. When the brass rail is not available, get one foot on any raised object: the bottom of a desk or the seat of a chair. NEVER maintain a stooped forward position when standing.

Lifting

Ideally you should not lift anything heavier than 15 lb while your back is sore and ideally you should not lift anything heavier than 50 lb for 6 months. When lifting something off the floor, bend the hips and knees keeping the spine straight, hold the object as close to the body as possible, then get up keeping the spine straight.

NEVER bend over to lift something off the ground with the knees straight.

NEVER hold anything weighing more than 15 lb more than 2 ft from the body.

NEVER lift anything over 20 lb above shoulder level.

Table 9.3. Instructions for Female Patients on Flexion Routine

General Observations

Whenever possible, sit down. Sit with the knees higher than the hips. The best way of doing this is to sit with the feet on a footstool. If no footstool is available, then cross the legs. Never sit with the legs out straight.

Don't reach.

Don't lift weights above the head.

Don't stoop.

Don't move furniture by pulling it in front of you.

Don't push windows up.

Don't put on weight.

Don't get overtired.

Don't maintain any one position for a prolonged period.

Sleeping

The mattress should be firm. If the mattress is soft, a board should be placed underneath it. Sleep on your side with your hips and knees bent.

Sitting

When driving a car the seat should be as close to the steering wheel as possible, thereby flexing the knees and hips. When riding in a car as a passenger, you should put a pillow behind your back so that you sit forward in the seat, again flexing the knees and hips. Whenever possible throughout the day, you should sit down with your knees higher than your hips in the "lazy boy" position.

Getting Up from Sitting

It is important not to arch the back on the act of getting up from sitting. Move to the front of the chair and stand up, keeping your back straight. Use your hands to help you if necessary.

Standing

The best way to stand it to adopt the posture commonly seen in a hotel: one foot on the ground and one foot on the brass rail. When the brass rail is not available, get one foot on any raised object: a footstool, the bottom of a desk, or the rung of a chair. NEVER maintain a stooped forward position when standing.

Lifting

Ideally you should not lift anything heavier than 10 lb while your back is sore and ideally you should not lift anything heavier than 20 lb for 6 months.

NEVER bend over to lift something off the ground with the back straight.

NEVER hold anything weighing more than 10 lb more than 2 ft from the body.

NEVER lift ANYTHING above shoulder level.

Housework

Equipment. All equipment should have long handles so that you do not have to stoop too much.

Vacuuming. The vacuum should be pushed with short sweeps rather than long lunges. Do not try to vacuum the whole house at once.

Kitchen. Never reach for objects from high shelves. Rearrange your kitchen so that articles which are in daily use are on the first shelf above counter level. When you have to stand for any length of time (ironing or at the kitchen sink), stand with one foot on a box 9 inches high. Use this box as a step to reach for articles above shoulder level. When getting articles out of cupboards underneath the counter level, bend your hips and knees, squat down keeping your back straight. Never stoop forward with the knees straight to reach for anything out of these low cupboards.

Table 9.3 (continued)

Laundry. When carrying laundry it is best to carry the clothes in a small basket held against one side. Never carry a heavy laundry basket in front of you. It is better to make several trips rather than to stagger once under an enormous load.

Stairs. Avoid as far as possible going up and down stairs. Do all the housework you have to do upstairs and then leave it for the day.

Bedmaking. You have to stoop forward when tucking in sheets and this will aggravate your back pain. When your back pain is severe, if you cannot persuade some other member of the family to do this chore, the only way you can tuck in the sheets in comfort is to get on your hands and knees.

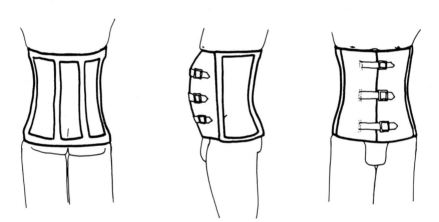

Fig. 9.14. A rigid spinal brace with posterior and side steels and a firm abdominal binder.

PSYCHOGENIC MAGNIFICATION OF DISABILITY

The chronic mildly depressed, the overwrought, the disconsolate, the weary, and the defeated patients have moved into third gear and have no drive to fight their way through their discomforts and, indeed, many have no apparent reason to do so. In these patients, if you are satisfied that, despite the psychogenic magnification of symptoms, they do indeed have an organic basis for pain, then you must develop a planned form of approach to their management.

The first thing you must accept is the fact that these patients give in readily to pain. In many this is due to a fear that any increase in pain signifies increasing damage to the spine, thereby decreasing their chances of recovery. Their disability is compounded by apprehension and misapprehension, and you must deal firmly with both. You must take time to explain that hurting and harming are not synonymous. You must make sure that they understand that an increase in discomfort does not mean that they have damaged their back. You must convince them that the only way they can really damage their spine is by sitting around doing nothing. You must get them to accept a measure of pain on activity and, indeed, recognize it as an index of cure.

Some are sensory weaklings and, despite your evangelical approach to the problem, they are defeated, deflated, and depressed by daily discomforts. You must mollify the discomfort by analgesics in order to push the patients into exercises and to stimulate increased activities. In any chronic pain syndrome there is grave danger in prescribing analgesics on demand, and in the emotionally destroyed this danger is of greater proportions. Analgesics should never be given on demand. The patients must never be permitted to pop pills for pain, to swallow their soreness away. They must be given analgesics on a time-dependent basis and the dosage, which should be more than adequate at the outset, should be gradually decreased without the patient's knowledge. The best way to do this is to give the analgesic in syrup form. For example, codeine can be made into a syrup containing 5 mg per ml. For 2 days before starting an exercise program, they should take 10 ml three times a day and then continue on the exercise program. If this is sufficient analgesia to get them started, they should then be allowed to finish 500 ml. When the prescription is renewed, it should contain only 4 mg per ml; the next 500 ml, 3 mg per ml; and so on, until the patient is taking just pure syrup at which time the dosage rate and quantity can be decreased.

By employing this technique the analgesic support can be decreased without the patient feeling deprived and, at the same time, if it is apparent to the physician that the rate of decrease of dosage is too rapid, the quantity of codeine in each milliliter can be increased in the next prescription, without the patient's knowledge and, thereby, without causing the patient alarm and despondency.

Unless you have a firm grasp and understanding of the underlying psychological problem, unless you have considerable knowledge of the posology, the complications, and the rapid changes in the forms of psychotropic medication available, do not play with them. You cannot give a patient a chemical vacation from his anxieties. If psychotropic medications are an essential part of treatment, they must be given solely by a physician versed in the technique of titrating these drugs against the patient's needs.

Unfortunately, one has to recognize and accept the fact that our present society is orientated to prescription drugs and otherwise. Some patients demand tranquilizers. If you feel you must give a patient a tranquilizer, then be honest about its purpose. Never slip a patient a pill with the dishonest notion that it is going to take the "spasms" away. If the patient troubles you that badly, take the tranquilizer yourself. Stick with simple medications such as chlordiazepoxide and sodium amobarbital. Stay away from diazepam because of the depressive effects after long term use.

Most of these patients need a rest in the day, not so much a physical rest, but a respite from the petty yet overpowering demands of daily living. The best way to prescribe this is by suggesting that they take a hot bath everyday for 1 hour. In the North American continent the bathroom is the only room in which you can shut yourself away for 1 hour without being thought peculiar. This intermittent daily convalescence is indeed extremely helpful for this group of patients.

The importance of recognizing emotional factors and their role in the constitution of the disability is of such importance that it has already been alluded to many times. It is discussed again when the failures following spinal surgery are described. I do not apologize for this deliberate repetition. Consideration of the emotional health of the patient is of paramount importance in the management of chronic low back pain and cannot be overly emphasized.

THE CERVICOLUMBAR SYNDROME

Symptomatic degenerative disc changes are most commonly seen in the lower lumbar spine. Occasionally the changes are multisegmental and involve the whole lumbar spine, and on occasion the changes are multifocal involving both the lumbar spine and the cervical spine. It is to this latter group that the term "cervicolumbar syndrome" has been applied. Commonly, the degenerative changes in the cervical spine are not symptomatic at the time that the patient is seen in regard to low back pain, or else the symptoms are relatively minor and the patient does

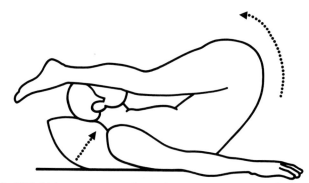

Fig. 9.15. With kick-up exercises, the patient may put a severe flexion strain on the neck, particularly if the neck is not supported by a pillow.

not feel them worthy of mention. As part of conservative treatment, the patient may be given sit-up or kick-up exercises. Sit-up exercises can place a severe extension strain on the neck, and in kick-up exercises the patient may injure the neck by straining or by overflexing (fig. 9.15).

As a result of the exercise program, the previously asymptomatic disc changes in the neck may become painful and may indeed constitute a significant continuing disability.

If a lumbosacral fusion is undertaken in such a patient, the hyperextended, rotated position of the neck adopted during the course of surgery may leave the patient subsequently with intractable cervicobrachial pain.

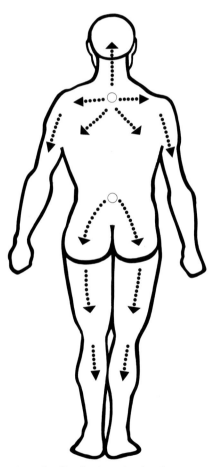

Fig. 9.16. Diagram to show the distribution of pain when symptoms are derived from degenerative disc disease in the cervical spine and the lumbar spine simultaneously. This gives rise to the unbelievable picture of total body pain.

If, when the patient is first seen, symptoms are derived from the degenerative changes in both the cervical and lumbar spines, the patient presents the almost unbelievable picture of "total body pain," pain in the neck radiating to the occiput, to both shoulders, and maybe down the arms. In addition, these patients may have pain radiating to the chest. The lumbar disc changes result in low back pain frequently associated with referred pain to one or both legs (fig. 9.16). It is little wonder, when confronted with such a picture, that the physician is defeated and examination and treatment tend to be perfunctory.

The importance of this syndrome is the awareness of its existence. Before suggesting sit-up or kick-up exercises for the treatment of low back pain, the patient should be specifically asked if he has any pain in his neck, shoulders, or arms. The neck should be examined carefully with particular attention being paid to the first sign of symptomatic cervical disc degeneration, namely, painful limitation of extension of the neck. If there is any suggestion of cervical disc degenerative changes in such patients, then the exercise program should be conducted with the patient's neck protected with cervical ruffs.

When the patient complains of what appears to be total body pain, the possibility of a cervicolumbar syndrome should be considered and its probability assessed by careful examination of both the cervical and lumbar spines. Admittedly, many of these patients are emotionally disturbed, but the emotional disturbance may be secondary to this irksome burden of pain. It is often wise to put the patient on a short course of adequate analgesia with mild sedation for a week, to allow the discomfort to subside, and then to re-examine the patient's clinical picture. There is no reason why simultaneous treatment for both the cervical disc changes and the lumbar disc changes should not be performed.

OPERATIVE TREATMENT

Spinal fusion as treatment of low back pain is rarely indicated. Nearly every back pain due to degenerative disc disease will settle to a tolerable level if the stress is taken off the spine by weight loss, strengthening of the abdominal muscles, the temporary use of a spinal support, and modification of activities occasionally involving a change of employment.

A spinal fusion may be considered in those instances in which an emotionally stable patient is unable, or is unwilling, to restrict work and pleasure activities or when, despite doing so, is still disabled by recurrent episodes of incapacitating low back pain.

The word "considered" is used advisedly. After admission to hospital,

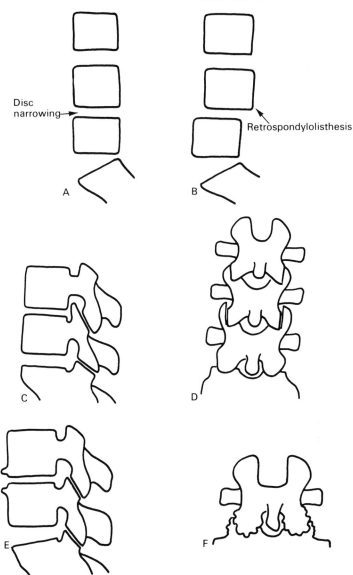

Fig. 9.17. Common x-ray changes seen with advancing disc degeneration: *A*, disc narrowing; *B*, retrospondylolisthesis; *C*, subluxation of the posterior joints revealed on the lateral view by virtue of the fact that the tip of the superior articular facet lies above a line drawn along the discal border of the vertebral body and extended posteriorly (the joint body line); *D*, subluxation of the posterior facets revealed on the anteroposterior view by the fact that the tip of the superior articular facet approaches the base of the transverse process of the vertebra above; *E*, traction spurs; and *F*, degenerative changes involving the posterior joints, recognized on x-ray by the gross irregularity in the outline of these joints.

two things must be assessed in greater detail: first, the patient who has the backache and, second, the backache the patient has.

In the natural history of degenerative disc disease, the L5–S1 disc is usually the first to be involved, followed subsequently by changes in the L4–L5 disc. Clinical experience has shown that the degenerative changes in the lumbosacral disc are self-limiting and rarely give rise to prolonged symptoms. The L4–L5 disc is the "backache disc" and a single segment L5–S1 fusion is rarely indicated.

Usually, by the time surgical intervention is considered, there are recognizable changes on x-ray: disc narrowing, retrospondylolisthesis, the traction spur, the Knuttson phenomenon, posterior joint subluxation, etc. (fig. 9.17). On occasion, the radiological changes are equivocal. It would be indefensible to perform a fusion without evidence of the offending site. This is one of the rare indications for diagnostic discography or, more accurately, discometric assessment.

Discography involves introducing a needle under x-ray control into the nucleus of an intervertebral disc and injecting contrast material. With the patient prone on the x-ray table, 20-gauge 3-inch needles are used to

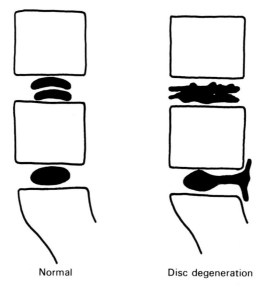

Normal   Disc degeneration

Fig. 9.18. Discography. With normal discs, the injected dye remains confined within the nucleus. The dye may present a spherical or bilobular appearance. When degenerative changes have taken place, the injected dye spreads throughout the disc and into the annulus. On occasion, it may be seen to spread posteriorly and run vertically underneath the posterior longitudinal ligament. This latter appearance, however, does *not* denote the presence of a disc rupture.

penetrate the interspinous ligament and the ligamentum flavum. Through these needles, 24-gauge 6-inch needles are placed through the dura into the disc and are advanced to the middle of the nucleus pulposus. The exact site of the tip of the needle is identified by x-rays taken in two planes. A water-soluble contrast material is then injected. If the disc is normal, the injected contrast material is confined to the nucleus. Although a normal disc offers considerable resistance to the injection, the resulting distension does not evoke a painful response. In the presence of disc degeneration, on the other hand, there is little or no resistance to the injection, the dye spreads diffusely through the disc, and the patient may experience pain.

At one time considerable significance was placed on the pattern of the injected dye (fig. 9.18). Increasing clinical experience has shown, however, that the only conclusion that can be drawn from the discographic pattern is either that the disc is normal or that it shows morphological evidence of degeneration. No statement can be made that the demonstration of morphological abnormality indicates that the disc injected is the source of symptoms.

Discography is an unreliable index of disc rupture or sequestration. The incidence of falsely positive and falsely negative results is very high. *The most important and most reliable finding on discography is the production or absence of pain on injection.*

The injection of a normal disc is painless. The injection of a degenerate disc may also be painless but, if the degenerative changes are symptomatic, distention of the disc reproduces the patient's clinically experienced symptoms.

The presence or absence of pain on distention of the disc is the important finding and the test is more accurately described as a "discometric assessment."

If this fact is acknowledged, discography is of greater value if the discs are injected first with saline. In contrast to the injection of radiopaque iodine compounds, the pain produced in a symptomatic degenerate disc on the injection of saline is of short duration. This short duration of pain is of importance, because it does not cloud and confuse the results of subsequent injection of other discs. Moreover, because of the low intensity and short duration of the discomfort produced, it permits the examiner to repeat the injection when necessary, to enable the patient to compare the pain with the clinically experienced symptoms.

The injection of contrast material is, however, an important integral part of the procedure. A very small quantity (0.5 ml) should be injected after the insertion of the needle to confirm the fact that the point of the needle is, indeed, lying in the center of the nucleus. At the conclusion of the procedure, dye should be injected to demonstrate the morphological pattern of the disc, thereby providing documentary evidence of a normal disc or a painless disc degeneration.

It must be remembered that lumbosacral disc degeneration, by itself, is very rarely the cause of long standing low back pain. When the degenerative changes revealed on straight x-rays of the lumbar spine appear to be confined to the lumbosacral disc, the L4–L5 disc must be checked carefully. Dynamic x-rays taken in flexion and extension may give evidence of abnormal movement at this segment. The straight x-rays may also give evidence of segmental instability in the form of a traction spur or the presence of a Knuttson phenomenon of air in the disc. Sometimes the earliest radiological evidence of disc abnormality is the radiological demonstration of posterior joint subluxation. Even in the absence of any radiological changes, the symptomatic health of the L4–L5 disc must be checked by discography. In the vast majority of such patients, the injection of the L4–L5 disc will reproduce the clinically experienced symptoms, and in such cases the surgeon knows that the L4–L5 segment must be included in the fusion mass.

Even if discography at the L4–L5 segment reveals a normal disc, it is not safe to presume that the presence of unequivocal radiological changes at the lumbosacral segment indicate that the L5–S1 disc is the source of pain. A single segment L5–S1 fusion is only justified in those patients in whom discography at L4–L5 is painless and a discogram at L5–S1 reproduces the clinically experienced symptoms. This is very unusual.

It is understandably tempting when the degenerative changes are confined to the L4–L5 segment to carry out an L4–L5 single segment fusion. Good results have been reported when an L4–L5 fusion has been combined with an L4–L5 discectomy. However, it must be admitted that an L4–L5 fusion may not have been necessary in these instances and a discectomy alone may have been enough to relieve the patient of his symptoms. Recurrence of symptoms is very common when an L4–L5 floating fusion is carried out for backache only. It is much safer, therefore, to extend the fusion down to the sacrum.

An L4–L5 fusion must never be performed unless the discs above are normal on discography. It has frequently been stated that a fusion, by applying excessive and unusual loads to the spine, precipitates degenerative changes at the segment above. However, in the balance of probabilities, in such instances degenerative changes were probably present at the segment above the fusion prior to operation even though not readily recognizable on standard radiographic examination. Since we have routinely used discometric analysis of the state of the disc above the proposed site of fusion, this complication has rarely been seen. This fact should give some confidence to the surgeons who feel that discography by itself may result in degenerative disc changes. If discography damaged the disc we should be seeing now, in our series, more patients with a damaged disc segment above the fusion, damage caused by the discography. This has not occurred.

It was stated at the beginning of this chapter that if, despite a course of adequate conservative treatment, the backache from which the patient was suffering significantly interfered with his capacity to do his work or his ability to enjoy himself in his leisure hours, he should be admitted to hospital for consideration of spinal fusion. The patient at this point in time must be warned that further investigations in hospital may reveal that spinal fusion is inadvisable because the more detailed analysis might demonstrate factors that would militate against a successful outcome.

The first and probably most important of such factors is reassessment of the patient as a whole, his personality, the workload he will face, and his physical condition, general and specific.

The extent of the degenerative changes in the lumbar spine has a profound influence on the results that can be reasonably anticipated. Although a gratifying result can be expected from an L4 to sacrum fusion, if the fusion must be extended cranially 2 inches to incorporate a degenerate L3–L4 segment, the success rate drops precipitously. There are two reasons for the evil connotation of the "terrible 2 inches," the three-segment fusion.

First, the incidence of pseudarthrosis is far greater; and, second, in a young or middle-aged person, the presence of symptomatic degenerative changes involving three segments generally indicate multifocal changes with a structurally inadequate spine. Even if the L2–L3 disc is shown to be normal on discometric analysis, it may, and frequently does, break down later. Many of these patients will also develop mirror image symptomatic degenerative changes in the cervical spine.

It is important, therefore, that prior to admission the patient is fully aware of the fact that careful appraisal of the mechanical integrity of the spine as a whole may result in the surgeon advising against spinal fusion. A three-segment fusion should only be carried out if the patient is emotionally stable and has a normal or high I.Q. The patient should be of normal weight and well muscled, and must have the opportunity of returning to light work. Moreover, he must be willing to accept the possibility of a second operation if a pseudarthrosis occurs.

Many surgeons feel that patients over 60 have reached an age of congratulation rather than operation. However, these are the only patients who do well with a spinal fusion for multicentric disc degeneration. This apparent paradox is due to the fact that the results of spinal fusion depend not only on the personality of the patient and the changes that have taken place in the spine, but they depend also on the demand that the patient will subsequently place on his spine. This group of patients does not ask very much. They cannot fully enjoy their retirement because they cannot sit in comfort to enjoy a game of bridge; they cannot play with their grandchildren; they cannot play golf; they cannot even sit through a play or movie at the theater. Although the pain is not excruciating or incapacitating, their backache is a bothersome burden. An interfacet fusion from L1 to the sacrum will make these people your most grateful patients.

It is essential that before any surgery the patient be made fully aware of the prolonged nature of the convalescence. The graft is rarely fully incorporated under 9 months. Sedentary workers and housewives may return to their duties with some persisting discomfort in 6 weeks. Patients whose jobs require prolonged standing, climbing stairs, walking, repetitive bending, and stooping rarely return to work in under 6 months. Heavy workers will take 1 year. None will really experience the full benefit of the operative procedure until about 1 year to 18 months following surgery.

Unless the patient is fully aware of the time involved and is prepared for it, the operation may lead to financial disaster. These points are particularly applicable when considering spinal fusion in the injured workman.

Operative techniques are the concern of the individual surgeon and are not dealt with here in any detail. Certain principles, however, are briefly discussed.

The modifications of the technique for spinal fusion initially described by Hibbs and Albee are legion, but in brief, they consist of corticocancel-

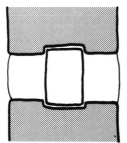 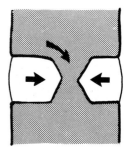

Fig. 9.19. A strut of cancellous bone placed across a disc space is infiltrated by fibrous tissue derived from the disc remnants before new bone, originating from the vertebral bodies, can replace the dead bone in the graft.

lous grafts wired to or wedged between the spinous processes, reinforced with or replaced by multiple bone chips, sometimes additionally stabilized with a temporary fixation afforded by interspinous plates, interlaminar rods, or facet screws. Internal fixation, however, only affords temporary stability.

In the 1950's with increasing surgical skills due largely to improved techniques of anesthesia, many surgeons, with thoughtless boldness, engaged in frontal assaults on the lumbar spine for degenerative disc disease. However, the initial wave of enthusiasm has now largely receded for several reasons. Apart from the operative hazard of damage to major vessels, unless a massive graft is employed to replace all the excised disc, a pseudarthrosis is likely to occur because it is easier for fibrous tissue derived from the remnants of the disc to invade the graft than it is for bone to grow from one vertebral body to the other (fig. 9.19).

Cortical grafts inhibit the invasion of fibrous tissue, and fibular strut grafts are best suited for interbody fusion. To ensure solid bony fusion, a massive amount of donor bone must be employed with the attendant problems of "donor site pain."

Anterior spinal fusion should be reserved as a salvage procedure.

Para-articular or intertransverse fusions present several advantages:

1. There is a continuous bed to which the graft may be applied (fig. 9.20).

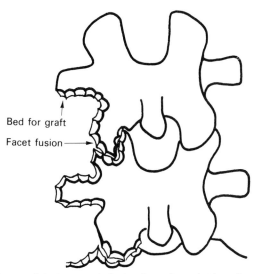

Bed for graft

Facet fusion

Fig. 9.20. When an intertransverse fusion is performed, there is a continuous bed of cancellous bone to which the bone graft can be applied. In addition to this, the intertransverse fusion can be combined with a facet fusion.

2. The technique permits intra-articular fusion or facet fusion. It has long been established that the achievement of facet fusion is mandatory for the success of the extensive fusions performed for scoliosis.
3. The fusion mass lies nearer the axis of movement.
4. The graft does not extend medial to the facets and the danger of an iatrogenic spinal stenosis, seen on occasion with routine posterior fusions, is thereby obviated.
5. The area of contact with the most superior vertebrae is greater than with the conventional posterior fusion and the likelihood of pseudarthrosis at this level is thereby decreased.

It is very difficult to assess the failure or success of a procedure such as a spinal fusion. If, in the reviews, subjective results are compared, many factors enter into the assessment of a patient. Even if x-ray results are compared, it is difficult to be sure whether a pseudarthrosis is present. However, in an attempt to assess the comparative success of anterior, intertransverse, or posterior fusions, a selected group of patients was studied. The patients were those in whom a double segment fusion of L4 to the sacrum was carried out for degenerative disc disease. None of the patients had ever been subjected to any previous surgery, and the operations were never combined with laminectomy and discectomy. The operative procedure was performed in each instance by the same surgeon. Lateral stress films were studied 2 years after surgery. Although it is acknowledged that there are many sources of error in assessing the incidence of pseudarthrosis from lateral stress films, it was presumed that this error would be equally distributed throughout the whole series studied, and therefore, the series would indeed by comparable (table 9.4). It can be seen from the analysis of this review that the results of intertransverse fusions compared very favorably with the results of other techniques.

The poor results of spinal fusion may be considered as stemming from three sources: the patient, the spine, and the surgeon.

The Patient. Good results are rarely achieved in the emotionally unstable patients with a low I.Q., heavy laborers with no alternate mode of employment, the obese, and the patients who are unable or unwilling

Table 9.4. Results of a Series of Patients Undergoing Double Segment Fusion

Type of Operation	No. of Cases	Pseudarthrosis	Percentage
Anterior interbody fusion	54	16	30
Posterior fusion	174	30	17
Intertransverse fusion	138	10	7

to accept a temporary change in life style. Every attempt should be made to avoid spinal fusion in the fat, flabby, fussed, and fearful.

The Spine. It is dangerous to operate on a spine without irrefutable evidence of the involved segments. Carrying out a spinal fusion in people whose spine shows multicentric disc degeneration is just patching an old coat, and good results cannot honestly be anticipated.

The Surgeon. The surgeon may be responsible for a bad result not only because of poor technique but probably more importantly and more commonly because of selection of the patient. The results of spinal fusion are usually disappointing in the presence of financially supported ill health or in those patients with a gross psychogenic magnification of symptoms, regardless of the underlying pathology.

The best results of spinal fusion are seen in the treatment of spondylolisthesis in the young and in the emotionally stable, financially secure, and physically fit housewife of 40 with degenerative disc disease involving the L4–L5 segment.

Spinal fusion for disc degeneration is not commonly indicated. The emotionally stable, intelligent patient can usually keep this self-limiting condition under control with slight modification of his daily rounds, and the emotionally fragile are rarely helped by this surgical exercise.

CHAPTER 10

Disc Degeneration with Root Irritation

"Thou cold sciatica, cripple our senators and make their limbs halt as lamely as their manners."

—W. Shakespeare

A patient with a mechanical compression of a lumbar nerve root will present with the complaint of sciatic pain with or without associated pain in the back. However, it cannot be too strongly emphasized that the mere complaint of pain in the leg does not indicate, by itself, root irritation or root compression. Any painful lesion in the lumbosacral region may give rise to pain referred down the leg in sciatic distribution.

This referred or "reflex" pain has the same neurophysiological basis as the referred pain to the shoulder associated with gallbladder disease and the referred pain down the arm associated with myocardial infarcts.

Referred sciatic pain derived from mechanical insufficiency of the lumbar spine is rarely experienced below the knee: it is not associated with paresthesia and there is no evidence of root tension, as reflected by limitation of straight leg raising or the presence of a positive bowstring sign.

In chapter 6 dealing with the pathogenesis of symptoms associated with degenerative disc disease, the pathological processes giving rise to root compression were described. The following discussion of the clinical features of lumbar root compression is confined to describing the symptoms and treatment of the two most common groups seen in clinical practice: disc rupture and the bony root entrapment syndromes.

DISC RUPTURES

Clinical Picture

Although most patients will try to remember some traumatic episode precipitating the attack, in the majority the symptoms will arise with minimal provocative incident. "I just bent down to tie my shoes,

Doctor." "I was pushing the lawn mower." "I got up out of my chair to turn off the TV." The onset is frequently dramatic. "I was seized with pain and couldn't move at all."

The symptoms may present in four ways: backache only, sciatica only, backache and sciatica, cauda equina compression.

It is difficult to differentiate the group of patients presenting with backache only from the acute episodes of back pain associated with posterior joint strain or subluxation. In some, however, despite the lack of pain radiating down the leg, on examination the patient demonstrates a marked limitation of straight leg raising. Even so, these patients should be treated by the method previously described for an acute posterior joint strain associated with segmental instability. *A manipulation, however, should not be attempted if there is any evidence on examination of root tension.*

Once the acute symptoms have abated, these patients have a regrettable propensity to recurrent attacks. The likelihood of a further episode can be lessened if the patient adheres to the rules of spinal hygiene and assiduously follows a flexion exercise program for a prolonged period of time.

More than half the patients will attribute their present attack to various forms of traumatic experience. This is retrograde rationalization on the part of the patient. Experimental studies and careful statistical analyses of case histories do not support the concept that direct trauma or sudden weight loading of the spine are the causal agents of disc rupture, although they may aggravate a pre-existing lesion. This aspect in the history becomes of importance when litigation or compensation is involved.

In a few patients sciatica is the only symptom. The majority start with back pain which subsequently radiates to the buttocks and then down the leg. Most patients report that as the sciatic pain increases the backache decreases in severity.

The history of pain is spondylogenic in character. The pain is aggravated by general and specific activities and is relieved by rest. Bending, stooping, lifting, coughing, sneezing, and straining at stool all intensify the pain. It is unreliable to attempt to identify the root involved by asking the patient to describe the anatomical distribution of the pain in the leg. It is rare for pain to radiate in a recognizable dermatome distribution.

Paresthesia, in the form of tingling, numbness, or a sensation of something trickling down the leg, is common and tends to confirm the diagnosis of root compression. It is interesting to note that although pain is more marked proximally (in the buttocks and upper thigh), numbness and tingling are more common in the leg and foot.

Unlike pain, paresthesia may be of localizing value. Numbness over the lateral side of the foot or in the sole of the foot suggests an S1 lesion; numbness extending to the dorsum of the foot and to the big toe, an L5 lesion; and numbness down the anteromedial aspect of the thigh is sometimes experienced with a lesion involving the fourth lumbar root.

Occasionally, the only symptom may be numbness of the foot and in the lower leg. The numbness is often vaguely localized and may have a stocking-like distribution suggestive of a neuropathy. It is rare is such instances for the patient to present objective evidence of impaired sensation. Rarely, motor symptoms predominate. The patient's complaint may be of a foot drop with little or no sciatic pain. In such instances, however, beware of a tumor.

The posture is characteristic. The lumbar spine is flattened and slightly flexed. The patient often leans toward the side of his pain, and this list becomes more obvious if he tries to bend forward. The patient is more comfortable if he stands with the affected hip and knee slightly flexed. He walks in obvious discomfort, frequently holding his loin with his hand. His gait is slow and deliberate and is designed to avoid any unnecessary movement of his spine. With gross tension on the nerve root, the patient may not be able to put his heel to the ground and walks slowly and painfully on tiptoe. Sitting down and getting up takes every bit of courage the patient can muster.

Forward flexion may be permitted so that the hands reach the knees. If the examiner keeps his fingertips on the spinous processes, he can see that the lumbar spine hardly moves at all and that flexion occurs mostly at the hip joint. Limitation of flexion in such instances, therefore, is a result of root tension. Measuring forward flexion is, in reality, measuring straight leg raising with the patient in the erect position.

Extension is limited and in most instances the pelvis starts to rotate as soon as the patient attempts to lean backward.

Lateral flexion may be full and free, but in the presence of a sciatic scoliosis, lateral flexion toward the convexity of the curve is limited.

The phenomenon of sciatic scoliosis and the relief or aggravation of pain on lateral flexion have been attributed to the position of the protrusion in relation to the nerve root (fig. 10.1). However, this may be a simplistic observation in view of the fact that the sciatic scoliosis disappears on recumbency. This observation—the loss of lateral curvature of the lumbar spine on recumbency—differentiates the sciatic list from a structural scoliosis.

On further assessment of the degree of root involvement present, it is imperative to test specifically for root tension, root irritation, and impairment of root conduction. These are the cardinal signs of lumbar root compromise.

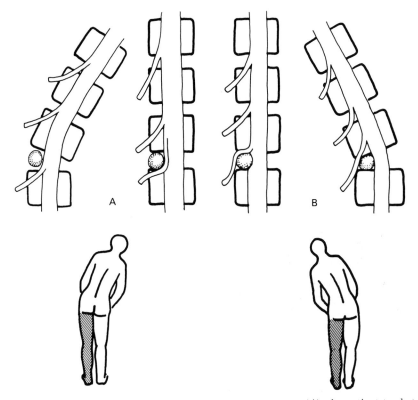

Fig. 10.1. When a disc protrusion is lateral to the nerve root (A), the patient tends to lean away from the side of the lesion to obtain relief of his discomforts. When, however, the disc herniation is in the axilla and lies medial to the root (B), the patient leans towards the side of the lesion to decrease the radicular pain.

Root Tension

The term "root tension" denotes distortion of the emerging nerve root by an extradural lesion. The two most useful tests of root tension are limitation of straight leg raising and the bowstring sign.

When testing straight leg raising, it is important not to hurt the patient. Never jerk the leg up in the air suddenly. The knee must be kept fully extended by firm pressure exerted by the examiner's hand. With the other hand over the heel, the examiner *slowly* raises the leg until leg pain or back pain is produced (fig. 10.2).

Two additional maneuvers are of vital importance to add significance to the finding of limitation of straight leg raising: (1) aggravation of pain by forced dorsiflexion of the ankle at the limit of straight leg raising (fig. 10.3); and (2) relief of pain by flexion of the knee. Sciatic pain is always relieved by flexing the knee.

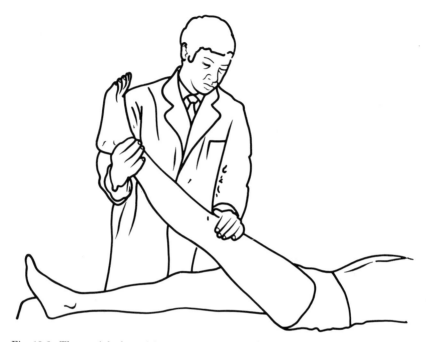

Fig. 10.2. The straight leg raising test. Note how the examiner maintains full extension of the knee joint while raising the leg.

If straight leg raising is permissible to 70° before pain is produced, the finding is equivocal, but below this level reproduction of pain on straight leg raising, aggravated by dorsiflexion of the ankle and relieved by flexion of the knee, is strongly suggestive of root tension. Reproduction of pain in the affected extremity by raising the unaffected leg is irrefutable evidence of root compression.

In patients in whom numbness in the foot is the predominant symptom, repetitive straight leg raising, i.e. "pumping of the leg," frequently intensifies the sensation of numbness.

The bowstring sign is the most important indication of root compression. The test has been described previously and is alluded to at this point briefly. The examiner carries out the straight leg raising to the point at which the patient experiences some discomfort. At this level, the knee is allowed to flex and the examiner allows the patient's foot to rest on his shoulder (fig. 10.4). The test demands sudden firm pressure applied to the popliteal nerve. This action may startle the patient enough to make him jump, and this jump may hurt. To prevent this, first of all, tell the patient you are just going to press firmly on the back of the knee. Apply firm pressure to the hamstrings; this won't hurt. Then move

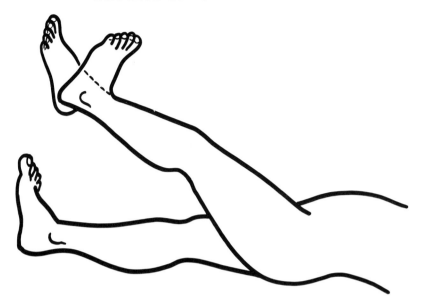

Fig. 10.3. At the limit of straight leg raising, if the ankle joint is forcibly dorsiflexed the patient may get an increase of the pain he experiences. This maneuver is particularly valuable in those patients in whom there is only minimal limitation of straight leg raising.

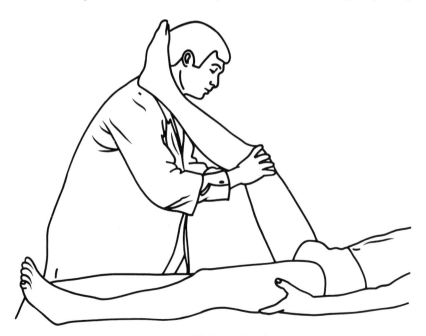

Fig. 10.4. The bowstring sign.

your thumbs over to the popliteal fossa, with the patient's knee held as straight as he will permit. Apply sudden firm pressure with your thumb over the popliteal nerve. Reproduction of pain in the leg or in the back is irrefutable evidence of nerve root compression. It is important to emphasize that if the test only produces local pain in the popliteal fossa, it is of no significance.

The demonstration of root tension is probably the single most important sign in the diagnosis of a ruptured intervertebral disc.

Root Irritation

Nerve root pain is probably the result of a combination of pressure and the inflammatory response to the prolapsed disc material. This "inflammatory response," this "radiculitis" has been loosely termed root irritation. Root irritation is an important factor in the demonstrated limitation of straight leg raising, and it would appear to be productive of peripheral muscle tenderness.

Such tenderness is not always present but, if demonstrable, is of value in localizing the level of root involvement. Frequently the calf is tender with S1 lesions, the anterior tibial compartment with L5 root involvement, and the quadriceps when the fourth lumbar nerve root has been compromised. The shin is the body image of the leg and very marked tenderness on palpating the subcutaneous surface of the tibia should warn the clinician that the patient has a large emotional component in his total disability picture. In the psychogenic regional pain syndromes, the patients frequently present skin tenderness with pain on just pinching the skin. Obviously, no meaningful statement can be made of the presence of deep muscle tenderness unless skin tenderness has been tested first.

It should be noted that the upper outer quadrant of the buttock is a tender area in most people with or without backache, and this area becomes increasingly tender in the presence of root irritation at any segment. It is of no localizing value. Patients with discogenic backache with root irritation may also present tenderness over the sacroiliac joint and down the course of the sciatic nerve.

Impairment of Root Conduction

The diagnosis of disc rupture is in no way dependent on the demonstration of root impairment as reflected by signs of motor weakness, changes in sensory appreciation, or reflex activity. However, the presence of such changes reinforces the diagnosis.

Sensory Impairment

The regions of sensory loss are reasonably constant (fig. 10.5). There appear to be areas more vulnerable than others. Loss of appreciation of

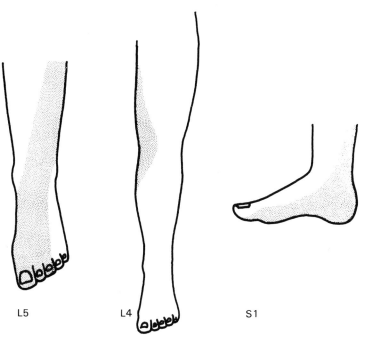

Fig. 10.5. Sensory innervation of the skin of the lower extremity.

pinprick is first noted in an S1 lesion below and behind the lateral malleolus and in an L5 lesion in the cleft between the first and second toe.

Sensory appreciation is a subjective response and, as such, may at times be difficult to assess. Certain precautions must be followed. Skin sensibility varies in different parts of the limb. Identical areas in each limb must be tested consecutively. The examination must be carried out as expeditiously as compatible with accuracy because the patient will soon tire of this form of examination and his answers may not be accurate.

When the skin is pricked with a pin, the physiological principle of recruitment is present. The overall sensory appreciation is dependent then not only on the action of a pinprick, but also on the total number of pinpricks experienced.

Patients over the age of 50 frequently demonstrate a delay in evaluating a sensory stimulus applied to the lower extremity. This is particularly applicable to the differentiation between hot and cold.

Motor Loss

Weakness of the gastrocnemii is best demonstrated by getting the patient to rise to tiptoe five or six times. The patient must be asked if it requires more effort to rise on tiptoe on the painful side. It is difficult to rise to tiptoe if the quadriceps are weak, and the physician must be wary of this before ascribing the difficulty of tiptoe raising to weakness of the calf muscles (fig. 10.6). Jumping on tiptoe may be painful and is not a good method of examination.

The power of the ankle dorsiflexors is best tested by applying full body weight to the dorsiflexed ankle (fig. 10.7). Testing the dorsiflexors by asking the patient to walk on his heels will only demonstrate marked weakness of this muscle group. Weakness of the flexor hallucis longus (S1) or weakness of the extensor hallucis longus (L5) is often the first evidence of motor involvement.

The gluteus maximus may become weak with lesions involving the first sacral nerve and may be demonstrated by the sagging of one buttock crease when the patient stands (fig. 10.8).

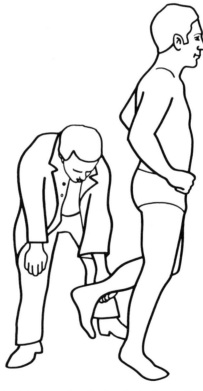

Fig. 10.6. It is important to recognize the fact that when trying to assess the strength of the gastrocnemius by asking the patient to rise on tiptoe, this action must be carried out repetitively and rapidly. The examiner is really attempting to assess fatigability of the muscle.

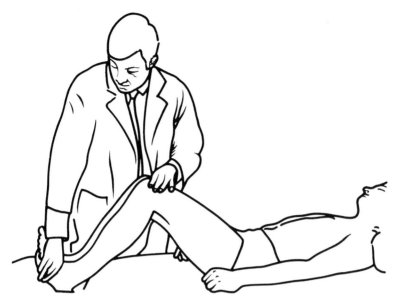

Fig. 10.7. When testing the strength of the dorsiflexors of the ankle, it is important to keep the knee flexed; otherwise this maneuver may aggravate the sciatic pain experienced by the patient and give rise to a false impression of weakness.

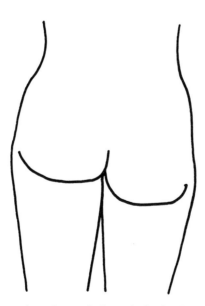

Fig. 10.8. The gluteus maximus is supplied mostly by S1. Lesions involving the first sacral root may cause weakness of the gluteus maximus which is apparent on examination by the sagging of one buttock crease.

Quadriceps weakness is seen with an L4 lesion and can be assessed by the examiner by placing his arm under the patient's knee and asking the patient to extend the knee against the resistance of the examiner's hand. However, this maneuver may produce pain, and a false impression of weakness is obtained. In such instances it is better to have the patient sitting over the edge of the table with his legs hanging free. The power of extension from 90° to 120° can be assessed without putting any stress on the sciatic nerve.

Muscle wasting is rarely seen unless the symptoms have been present for more than 3 weeks. However, the girth of the calf and the thigh should always be measured. This will act as a base line, on occasion, to assess progress of the lesion. It must be remembered that, if there is gross weakness of the gastrocnemii, the main venous pump of the affected extremity is no longer working, and these patients may indeed show some measure of ankle edema. The combination of calf tenderness due to S1 root irritation and the observation of a swollen ankle may give rise to the erroneous diagnosis of a thrombophlebitis. If this has not been noted preoperatively in patients who are subjected to operation, they may be started unnecessarily on a course of anticoagulants.

Changes in Reflex Activity

The ankle jerk may be diminished or absent with an S1 lesion. It is best tested with the patient kneeling on a chair. If the patient has suffered a previous attack of sciatic pain with sufficient compression of the first sacral nerve to knock out the ankle jerk, this rarely returns. The absence of an ankle jerk, therefore, may merely be a stigma of the previous episode of disc rupture, and the present attack may be due to a disc rupture at another level.

Scratching the sole of the foot, as in the plantar response, produces a reflex contraction of the tensor fascia femoris. This little known reflex is often lost with an S1 lesion.

With L4 and L3 lesions, the knee jerk may be diminished. Many other deep tendon reflexes can be tested; however, assessment of the reflexes mentioned has been of the greatest value in the routine clinical assessment of the clinical syndrome of the ruptured disc.

The common neurological changes are summarized in figure 10.9.

Radiographic Examination

The major value of x-rays of the lumbar spine in the routine assessment of a disc rupture is to exclude more serious pathology such as tumors or infections that may mimic the syndrome. X-rays are not of any localizing value. The demonstration of a narrowed disc space does not necessarily indicate that this represents the involved level.

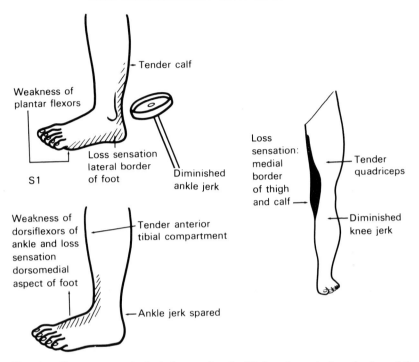

Fig. 10.9. Common neurological changes found with impairment of conduction of the lower lumbar nerve roots.

Myelography should only be employed if surgical intervention is considered. It should never be used as a routine diagnostic measure unless the clinical findings raise the possibility of a tumor.

Conservative Treatment

Treatment obviously varies according to the severity of the root compression and can best be considered under the following clinical syndromes: aggravating leg pain and incapacitating leg pain.

Aggravating Leg Pain

These are patients who after certain activities develop a dull, nagging sciatic pain that slows them down. The patients learn to recognize that if they do certain things their sciatica will flare up and they may have to give up playing golf or tennis, and they may markedly modify their work activities. Their pain is never sufficiently severe to stop them from getting on with their daily rounds, but it "bugs" them.

Theoretically, the best way to heal the underlying pathology would be to take all the mechanical loading off the spine by putting the patient to bed for 3 weeks. However, the physician is treating a patient, not a spine, and, with the type of symptoms presented, it would be unreasonable to expect the patient to follow this sort of advice. The same principles, therefore, must be followed as in the treatment of chronic symptomatic degenerative disc disease.

Unload the Spine. The following measures must be undertaken to take weight off the spine:

1. Loss of weight where indicated.
2. Modification of work and play activities: the flexion routine.
3. Increase of intra-abdominal pressure, temporarily by a corset, and permanently by building up the strength of the abdominal muscles. In the thin patients, the corset will not be of much value unless it is padded well in front to add direct pressure on the abdomen. Some of these patients are better treated with a thoracopelvic brace to protect the spine against unexpected jars and strains.
4. Physical rest until the pain starts to abate. The patient should spend the evenings in bed.

Anti-inflammatory Drugs. The sciatic pain is due in part to a perineural inflammatory response to the extruded disc material. In many instances, this inflammatory change can be decreased by anti-inflammatory drugs.

Analgesics. As in all chronic pain problems, analgesics must be given on a time-dependent basis, not on demand.

The majority get better in about 6 weeks. In a few, however, the pain persists to a degree that demands further attention. Before considering surgical intervention, two alternate methods of treatment can be considered: infiltration of the nerve root sleeve under x-ray control with hydrocortisone, or enzymatic dissolution of the disc by the intradiscal injection of chymopapain.

Incapacitating Leg Pain

When the pain is incapacitating in severity, the patient must go to bed. A plaster jacket has no role in treatment. The patient is allowed to move around in bed and assume whatever position he finds most comfortable. He may get up to use the toilet, using crutches if walking is difficult. After 48 hours most patients are relatively comfortable apart from sudden movements. Traction (either leg traction or pelvic traction) is only indicated if severe pain persists despite bedrest and analgesics. Traction does not help everyone, and its value should first be assessed by applying manual traction to the leg. If the patient feels better when you pull on his leg, the skin traction with a 10-lb weight will keep the patient more comfortable while in bed (fig. 10.10). Remember that traction is not

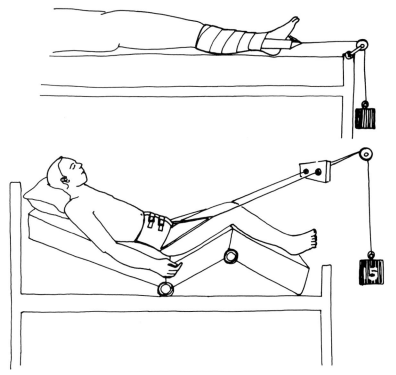

Fig. 10.10. Traction, either leg traction or pelvic traction, should only be continued if the patient experiences significant relief while the traction is being applied.

curative; its sole function is to decrease pain. It carries the occasional hazard of thrombophlebitis.

The patient should stay in bed until he has been relatively comfortable for 48 hours in his journeys to the toilet. The rate of improvement should not be assessed by testing straight leg raising daily. This gives rise to unnecessary discomfort and tends to alarm the patient. Once the patient is up and around, the routine treatment for chronic degenerative disc disease is instituted.

How long should the physician persist with bed rest as a form of therapy? Initially, when herniated discs were first described, many physicians demanded 6 weeks of complete bedrest. However, we must remember that 6 weeks in bed without any guarantee of recovery might be financially disasterous. I think that most would agree that the maximal time in bed that a surgeon can demand from a patient who has shown no improvement whatsoever is 3 weeks. With the introduction of chemonucleolysis, probably the intradiscal injection of chymopapain should be considered after 2 weeks of bedrest as the last resort of conservative therapy.

Preoperative Evaluation

The indications for operative treatment are now well established (table 10.1).

In the cauda equina syndrome with bladder and bowel paralysis, surgical decompression is imperative and urgent. Gross weakness of one muscle group, particularly the dorsiflexors of the ankle, or progressive weakness, despite bedrest, demands surgical relief.

In the absence of these absolute indications for surgery, the physician must consider carefully the question, "Why has conservative treatment failed?" "Is it because of the nature of the disc lesion?" "Have emotional factors led to an erroneous assessment of the patient's problem?"

If the physician has no doubt as to the physiogenic basis for the pain and is perfectly satisfied that conservative treatment has been adequately followed out, then surgical intervention is justified.

Radiographic Examination

Although x-ray examination of the back has but little value in the diagnosis of disc herniation, it plays a very important role in the preoperative assessment of the patient.

Anomalies of segmentation are common. The fifth lumbar vertebra may become assimilated with the sacrum (sacralization of L5) or the first sacral segment may be mobile (lumbarization of S1) resulting in six mobile lumbar vertebrae. The last mobile segment, therefore, instead of being L5-S1 may be at L4-L5 or at S1-S2.

Superficially, it would seem that this would not create any diagnostic difficulties and that the correct segmentation could be determined by counting down from the first lumbar vertebra. However, the 12th rib is frequently rudimentary or absent, and it is difficult to be sure whether the first vertebral segment in the lumbar spine is indeed L1 or whether it

Table 10.1. Indications for Laminectomy

---

1. ABSOLUTE
    A. Bladder or bowel paralysis (cauda equina syndrome)
    B. Marked muscular weakness
    C. Progressive neurological defect despite complete bedrest
2. RELATIVE
    A. Intolerable pain in an emotionally stable patient despite bedrest and traction
    B. Pain unrelieved by complete bedrest
    C. Recurrent episodes of incapacitating sciatica

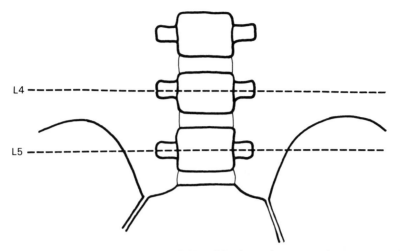

Fig. 10.11. With a normal anatomical disposition it can be seen on the anteroposterior x-ray that the transverse processes of L5 lie below the iliac crest whereas the transverse processes of L4 lie above the iliac crest.

is the 12th thoracic vertebra mimicking L1 because of the absence of a rib.

In an attempt to make an accurate numerical judgment of the segments of the lumbar spine without taking an x-ray of the whole vertebral column, the following points should be remembered. The transverse processes of L5 are below the level of the iliac crest. The transverse processes of the fourth lumbar vertebrae are above the level of the iliac crest (fig. 10.11). The transverse processes of the lumbar vertebrae tends to point cranially whereas the transverse processes of the 12th dorsal vertebra point caudally. Usually the third lumbar vertebra has the largest transverse processes (fig. 10.12). Using these criteria, with the normal anatomical configuration, if a rupture of the last mobile disc is indeed the L4-L5 disc, then the fifth lumbar root will be compromised, and if the last mobile disc is the S1-S2 disc, then the second sacral root will be involved (fig. 10.13).

Myelography

As mentioned previously, myelography has no place in the diagnosis of a disc herniation, but it is an essential facet of preoperative investigation. Myelography has two purposes: first, to rule out the remote possibility of a nerve root tumor masquerading as a disc, and second, to localize the site of herniation in relation to the lamina of the involved segment and thereby limit the extent of surgical exposure.

It is not the purpose of this text to discuss in detail the radiological

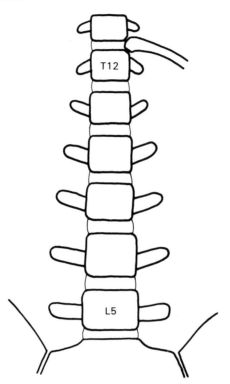

Fig. 10.12. The transverse processes of the lumbar vertebrae tend to point cranially whereas the transverse processes of the dorsal vertebrae point caudally.

changes that may be seen on myelography, but some general principles regarding the interpretation of myelograms are described.

The principle of myelography is to fill the subarachnoid space and the emerging nerve roots with a radiopaque fluid, usually referred to as a radiopaque dye. Space-occupying lesions, whether they be extra- or intrathecal, interfere with the flow of the injected dye, thereby localizing the site and demonstrating the size of the lesion. Diagrams of the myelographic defects of common lesions are shown in figure 10.14.

However, a significant lesion may be present without producing any myelographic defect under the following circumstances. If the lesion is very lateral, it will not encroach on the dural tube and will not create a flow defect. Similarly, defects may not be seen if the dural sac is narrow or if it does not extend caudally to the sacrum (fig. 10.15). The dural sac tapers as it approaches the sacrum, and for these reasons a falsely negative myelogram is most commonly seen at the lumbosacral junction.

A diffuse bulge of the annulus arising as a result of disc degeneration is most commonly encountered at L4-L5. This lesion, which is rarely associated with root compression, may produce an hourglass constriction of the myelographic oil column, giving rise to the erroneous impression of a bilateral disc herniation or a "central" disc (fig. 10.16). Of myelography, it can be said in general that false negatives are seen at L5-S1 and false positives at L4-L5.

Every clinician will agree that the decision to perform a laminectomy and discectomy must be based on a careful clinical appraisal of the patient. Most surgeons feel that a myelogram is an essential preoperative investigation. If, however, the myelogram does not show any abnormalities, then there are two schools of thought.

Some will persist with conservative treatment regardless of the

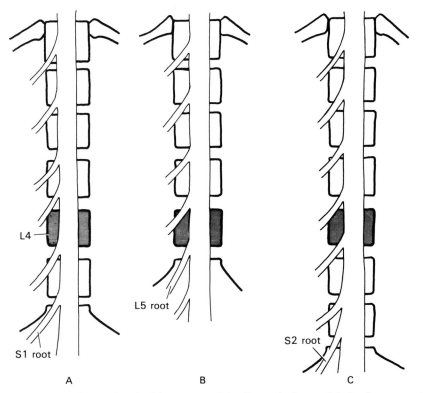

L4

L5 root

S1 root

S2 root

A   B   C

Fig. 10.13. The root involved by rupture of the disc at the last mobile lumbar segment will, of course, depend on the segmentation of the lumbar vertebral column. In the normal vertebral column with five mobile lumbar vertebrae (A), the first sacral root will be involved; when there is sacralization of the fifth lumbar vertebra (B), a disc rupture of the last mobile segment will compress the fifth lumbar nerve root; when there is lumbarization of the first sacral segment with six mobile lumbar vertebrae (C), then a rupture of the last mobile disc will involve the second sacral root.

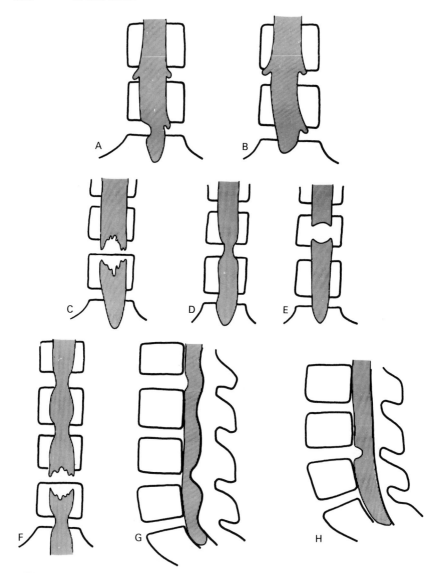

Fig. 10.14. Diagrammatic representation of commonly seen myelographic defects. *A,* Lumbo-sacral disc rupture with indentation of the oil column. *B,* Cut-off of the first sacral root sleeve due to a lateral disc rupture. *C,* Sequestration of a large fragment of disc material at the L4-L5 level. *D,* Annular constriction of the oil column at the L4-L5 level. This radiographic appearance is produced by a diffuse annular bulge of the L4-L5 disc and is *not* due to a bilateral disc protrusion. *E,* An intrathecal tumor will produce a characteristic defect delineated by a meniscus. Frequently, this defect is in relation to a vertebral body on x-ray, rather than to the disc space. *F,* Compression of the cauda equina from a posterior lesion such as a spinal stenosis may produce a complete block in the oil column on the anteroposterior view, but the true site of the lesion will be revealed by studying the lateral view (*G*) where it can be seen that there is a marked posterior indentation. *H,* Anterior indentations of the oil column are frequently seen on the lateral view, but these are rarely of clinical significance.

severity of the symptoms. This is scarcely justifiable because, as just stated, under certain anatomical conditions a large extradural lesion (such as a ruptured disc) can be present without producing any myelographic defect. If root compression is allowed to persist too long, it may eventually lead to perineural and intraneural fibrosis of the root: a condition that may give rise to prolonged significant disability, and

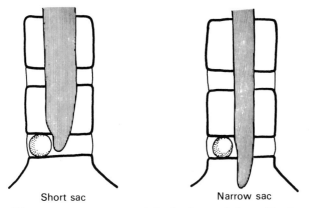

Short sac   Narrow sac

Fig. 10.15. Disc ruptures may occur at the lumbosacral disc without producing any myelographic defect whatsoever. This is particularly true in the presence of a short sac or a very narrow thecal sac.

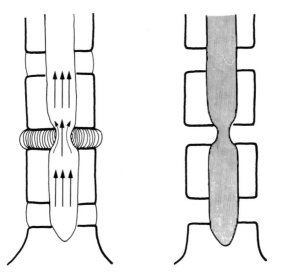

Fig. 10.16. A diffuse annular bulge produces a watershed effect. Because the column of the fluid in the theca flows more rapidly as it passes over the hump produced by the diffuse annular bulge, the increased rate of flow at this site will produce narrowing of the oil column. The resulting waisting at this level may give rise to the erroneous impression of a bilateral disc rupture.

which is almost impossible to treat by surgical techniques presently available.

Some surgeons, when faced with the problem of severe root compression without localizing neurological deficit, will, in the presence of a normal myelogram, be willing to widely explore the last three lumbar segments, the so-called "exploratory laminotomy."

An exploratory laminotomy, however, is not an innocuous procedure. At the conclusion of the operation, the rawed surface of the sacrospinalis is placed in intimate contact with the dura, and significant and symptomatic perineural and peridural fibrosis may result. It is advisable to keep the exposure as small as possible. To do this, it is important to localize the site of the lesion accurately before surgery. Other methods of investigation are available and if the myelogram is apparently normal, they should be employed.

Nerve Root Infiltration

If the involved nerve root is infiltrated with local anesthetic (2% lidocaine) at its point of emergence through the root canal, the sciatic pain experienced by the patient will be abolished. The technique of root sleeve infiltration is very easy at the L5-S1 foramen and above. With the patient lying on his side, an 18-gauge needle is inserted 12 cm from the midline and directed toward the foramen under image intensifier control. The patient should be well sedated because when the needle hits the root the patient experiences a sudden flash of pain down the leg. At this stage, 0.5 ml of an oil-soluble contrast material is injected into the root sleeve. If the root sleeve has been entered, the injected dye assumes a tubular configuration. If the root sleeve has not been entered, the dye diffuses in a circular fashion. After correct placement of the needle 1 ml of 2% lidocaine is injected.

The first sacral root is more difficult to inject. The patient is placed face downwards on the table, and the needle is inserted through the first dorsal sacral foramen to emerge through the first ventral foramen before the dye and the local anesthetic are injected (fig. 10.17). This is a much more difficult maneuver.

Abolition of leg pain following root sleeve infiltration convincingly demonstrates the site of the lesion.

Epidural Phlebography

The epidural veins are remarkably constant in their anatomical disposition (fig. 10.18). The anterior internal vertebral veins run vertically and lie in close apposition to the invertebral discs. A laterally placed disc rupture, not demonstrable on myelography, in a patient with

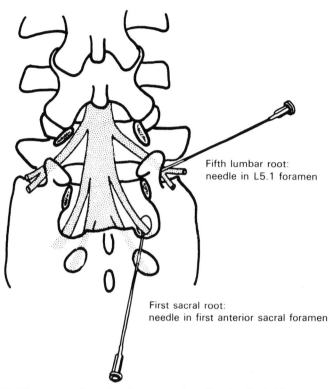

Fifth lumbar root:
needle in L5.1 foramen

First sacral root:
needle in first anterior sacral foramen

Fig. 10.17. Diagram to show the placement of needles for the infiltration of the fifth lumbar and first sacral nerve roots.

a short or narrow dural sac, will be demonstrated by the fact that the flow in the vertebral vein running over the disc protrusion will be interrupted (fig. 10.19).

The vertebral veins lying within the spinal canal communicate by the radicular veins with longitudinal venous channels lying immediately anterior to the transverse processes. These radicular veins run in close apposition to the nerve roots as they course through the intervertebral foramina. Because the nerve root sleeves do not fill well with the oil-soluble contrast materials commonly used for myelography, a routine myelogram will not demonstrate compression of a root within the foramen, but flow in the radicular veins may be interrupted.

The epidural veins can be outlined by the percutaneous catheterization of the femoral vein and advancement of the catheter into the external vertebral vein under x-ray control. With the vertebral venous plexus clearly outlined by the injection of contrast material, interruption of venous flow can be readily demonstrated.

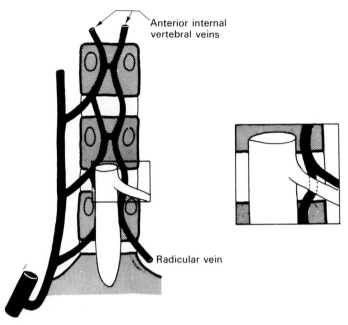

Fig. 10.18. Diagram to show the disposition of the anterior internal vertebral veins and the radicular veins. It can be seen that the anterior internal vertebral veins are closely apposed to the intervertebral disc and that the radicular veins cross the intervertebral disc accompanying the nerve roots as they emerge through the intervertebral foramina.

Electromyography

Evaluation of the electrical activity of muscles, either at rest or with contraction, may be used to localize the level of lumbar nerve root involvement. Healthy, normally innervated muscle is electrically "silent" at rest and the insertion of an electromyographic needle does not produce sustained electrical discharges. However, in the presence of a nerve root lesion, a series of involuntary electrical discharges can be recorded. These are characterized by a shortened potential and reduced amplitude (*fibrillation potentials*) or by altered wave forms (*positive waves*). The positive wave forms are only produced on needle insertion, but the fibrillation potentials can be recorded all the time.

On voluntary contraction of a normal muscle, the action potentials evoked are biphasic or triphasic in form. With partial denervation, the quantity of motor units recording is decreased and polyphasic waves are seen (fig. 10.20).

The paraspinal muscles are supplied by the posterior primary rami of the emerging lumbar nerve roots. In the electromyographic examination

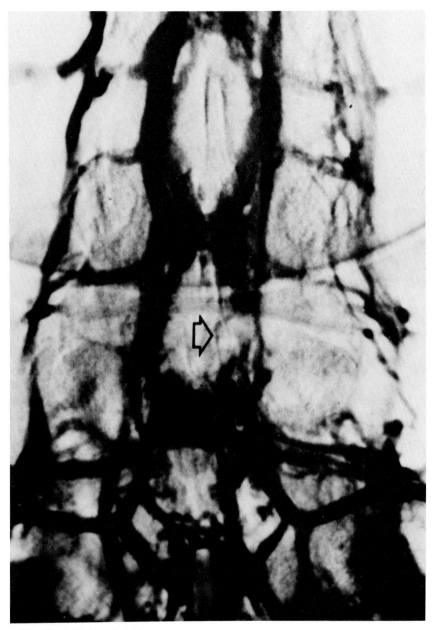

Fig. 10.19. Epidural phlebogram. In this phlebogram the anterior internal vertebral vein is occluded on one side as it crosses over the intervertebral disc. This is the classic radiological change associated with a disc rupture.

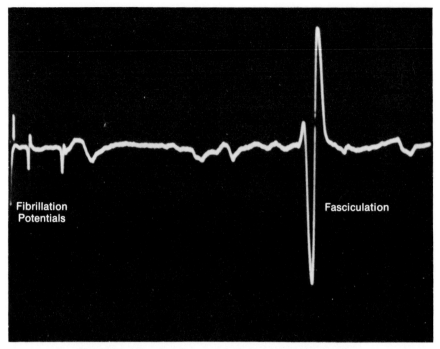

Fig. 10.20. A drawing of normal and abnormal EMG changes.

of a patient suffering from nerve root compression, the electrical activity of the paraspinal muscles at rest and on voluntary activity is observed. Lesions producing interference of root conduction will demonstrate the electromyographic changes described.

In addition to testing the paravertebral muscles, the muscles in the lower limbs innervated by the lumbar nerve roots must also be assessed. In S1 lesions the examination can be broadened to include the sensory limb of the sciatic nerve. It is possible to stimulate the afferent limb of S1 with an electrode in the popliteal fossa and to measure the time required to travel to the dorsal root, pass through the reflex arc, travel down the efferent limb, and eventually produce a contraction of the gastrocnemius. This is the Hoffmann reflex, sometimes referred to as the H-reflex. With S1 root involvement, the time between the sensory stimulus and the motor response will be prolonged, and the pattern of the evoked potential may be abnormal.

In summary, the major electromyographic changes associated with nerve root compression are fibrillation potentials and positive sharp waves at rest, and a decrease in the number of active potentials on voluntary activity associated with the presence of polyphasic waves. In

S1 lesions, a prolonged latency or absence of the H-reflex is of great diagnostic significance.

Electromyographic examination may demonstrate root lesions at several levels. This may be seen with spinal stenosis, but it is also seen in metabolic disorders such as diabetes and in subclinical neuropathies. Electromyography is of great value in the assessment of hysterical paralysis.

There is regrettable tendency when reporting the diagnostic accuracy of electromyography and myelography, to compare the two. They are not, however, alternative methods of examination; they should be used to supplement each other. Electromyography is able to localize specific root involvement, but does not give any information as to the site of the lesion or the nature of the lesion. Myelography, on the other hand, gives information in regard to the anatomical location of the lesion and the probable pathology.

Discography

When the technique of discography was originally introduced, it was hoped that the demonstration of posterior extravasation of dye from the disc would constitute an adequate radiological demonstration of a disc rupture. Clinical evaluation, confirmed by the examination of discs injected at autopsy, has failed to substantiate this initial hope. Small tears in the annulus commonly found in patients over 30 years of age permit posterior extravasation of the dye, even in the absence of a disc rupture. However, as mentioned in the section dealing with disc degeneration, some significance can be placed on the reproduction of clinically experienced symptoms on distending the disc. Reproduction of sciatic pain on injecting a disc is powerful evidence that the level of the disc rupture has been found.

Discography, however, remains the last resort of ancillary investigations under the following conditions: when the myelogram is negative; when the epidural phlebogram is difficult to interpret because the radiological pattern is obscured by retained contrast material in the dural sac; when root infiltration proves to be technically impossible; and when the findings on electromyography are equivocal. In such an unhappy, uncertain clinical situation, discography comes into its own.

Laminectomy

The operative technique of a laminectomy is a matter of individual preference and is not described here. However, certain principles applicable to whatever technique is employed are enumerated briefly.

When the patient is positioned the abdomen must be completely free in order to avoid compressing the vena cava which inevitably leads to congestion of the epidural veins. You can't be sure that you have completely released the nerve unless you can see it well and continuously. The occasional glance, as the sucker is plunged into the wound is not enough. Hemostasis must be maintained meticulously (fig. 10.21).

The nerve root must be identified, defined, and seen clearly before any incision is made into the disc. A grossly flattened nerve root may assume an appearance alarmingly similar to the posterior fibers of the annulus and may be incised in error.

The contents of the disc should be removed as completely as possible. The removal of degenerative disc material should be accomplished with a curette, never with biting forceps which carry with them the danger of penetration of the anterior fibers of the annulus and damage to the great vessels or ureters.

At the conclusion of disc enucleation, the root should lie free and it should be possible to displace it medially at least 1 cm with ease. If the root cannot be displaced, it must be followed throughout its course to its point of emergence from the foramen, if necessary, to demonstrate the cause of the tethering and to free it.

At the conclusion of the operation, the laminectomy defect must be covered with an impervious barrier such as Silastic or Gelfoam to prevent fibroblasts derived from the rawed surface of the sacrospinalis from invading the inevitable peridural hematoma and thereby producing a progressive peridural and periradicular fibrosis (fig. 10.22).

Following the operation, the patient must be given instructions as to how to protect his back for a period of time (table 10.2). For 6 months he should follow the rules of spinal hygiene as previously described for disc degeneration.

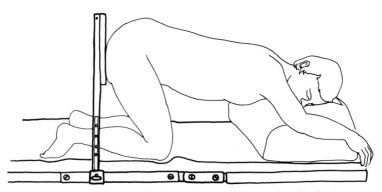

Fig. 10.21. Diagram of the modified knee-chest position employed in laminectomy. The use of a buttock rest and chest support enables the abdomen to lie free without any external pressure whatsoever.

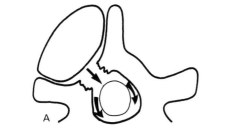

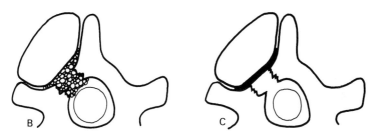

Fig. 10.22. At the conclusion of a laminectomy the rawed surface of the sacrospinales is placed against the laminotomy. This permits invasion of the peridural space by fibroblast derived from the sacrospinales (A). This fibrotic invasion can be inhibited by closing the bony defect with Gelfoam (B) or by the use of an interposition membrane (C).

Table 10.2. Patient Instructions Following Laminectomy

Following discharge from hospital your activities should be restricted in the following manner:

First week: Get up late; rest in the afternoon; go to bed early. May be driven in a car, but do not drive yourself. No lifting. May take shower or tub bath.

Second week: Increase activities within limits set by fatigue (women—light housework). Bed early. May drive own car.

Third week: May return to light work.

Fourth week: Normal activities except those which involve repetitive bending, rotation under stress, lifting more than 50 pounds as a straight lift or 20 pounds with the weight held at arm's length.

Eighth week: No restrictions.

It is quite common to get occasional twinges of pain in one or both legs and it is also common to have cramps in the calf particularly at night time. These are not of significance and will pass away by themselves.

If you had any degree of numbness or weakness before the operation, this may take several weeks to recover and return to normal state.

When activities are increased you are bound to get some aching in the back as the scar tissue is stretched. This need not cause any alarm and need not indicate any curtailment of activities. Backache of this type may last for 1 or 2 months.

There is an unresolved discussion as to whether laminectomy should be combined with a spinal fusion. This decision is largely based on the total clinical assessment of the patient. If the clinical story is of a single episode of severe sciatic pain with minimal backache, or repeated attacks in each of which the sciatic pain is much more severe than the associated backache, a discectomy alone is all that is required. If, however, the story is of repeated episodes of back pain gradually increasing in severity and finally culminating with episodes of backache associated with severe sciatic pain due to nerve root irritation, discectomy alone may possibly rid the patient of the sciatic pain, but more than likely he will be left with recurrent episodes of backache similar in character and severity to the episodes which incapacitated the patient in the past. In such instances, the problem is really one of mechanical instability of the spine, recently associated with a disc herniation. The treatment of choice is laminectomy and fusion. If a decision is made to fuse the spine, then the health of the disc above the proposed level of fusion must be assessed by discography. A fusion should only be carried out below a segment shown to be normal on discography; otherwise, the extra mechanical stresses imposed by the fusion may well accelerate the degenerative changes and these in turn may become symptomatic.

BONY ROOT ENTRAPMENT SYNDROMES

The pathological changes giving rise to constriction of a spinal canal (spinal stenosis) and bony compression of the emerging nerve roots are described in chapter 6.

Patients suffering from spinal stenosis may present with backache, backache and sciatica, or sciatica only. Clinical evaluation of patients with spinal stenosis supports the thesis that the complaint of radicular pain implies lateral or apophysial stenosis. The radicular pain may differ from the sciatic pain due to a disc herniation in that it can, on occasion, present a "claudicant" character being precipitated, aggravated, and progressively intensified by the act of walking. It differs from the claudicant calf pain of peripheral vascular insufficiency in that the pain is experienced first, and most severely, proximally in the limb. The increasing symptoms produced by continuing to walk frequently manifest themselves as paresthesia noted in the calf and foot and are often associated with the subjective sensation of weakness. Unlike the pain associated with vascular insufficiency, the claudicant radicular pain does not abate on standing still. The patient has to sit down or lie down to get relief.

Bony compression of an emerging nerve root does not invariably give rise to this claudicant type of pain. It may present simply as sciatica, being aggravated by general and specific activities. The clinical picture of bony root entrapment differs, however, in several aspects from the syndrome of a disc rupture.

The first important difference is the age incidence. Under 40 years of age, disc ruptures are by far the most common cause of radicular pain. Between the age of 40 and 50, bony root entrapments occur with equal frequency, but over 50 bony root entrapment syndromes are by far the most common source of root irritation.

Patients with bony root entrapment usually give a history of long-standing backache with a recent onset of sciatica. On examination, despite severe sciatic pain, one of the remarkable findings is the fact that straight leg raising is rarely significantly limited.

A true disc herniation with extrusion of nuclear material very rarely occurs at more than one segment. Apophysial stenosis, on the other hand, frequently involves several roots. Although a large central disc, a disc extruding laterally into the foramen, or a disc rupture in association with an anomaly of root emergence may involve more than one root, usually when there is clinical evidence of multiple root involvement, the probability of a bony root entrapment is much greater (fig. 10.23).

The changes seen in a routine x-ray of the lumbar spine are never of diagnostic significance in a ruptured disc. With root stenosis several characteristic changes may be recognized. The bony root entrapment syndromes are frequently associated with subluxation of the posterior

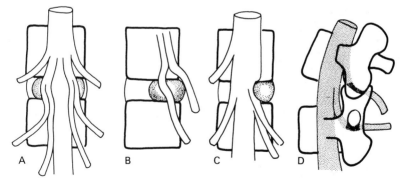

Fig. 10.23. A disc rupture usually involves one nerve root only. However, multiple nerve roots may be involved under the following circumstances: *A*, a central disc; *B*, a lateral disc compressing the nerve root that passes over it and compressing the nerve root that emerges through the foramen at this segment; *C*, an anomaly of root emergence with two nerve roots emerging through the same foramen. With this anatomical anomaly a disc rupture will, of course, compromise both these nerve roots as they cross over the disc.

Apophysial stenosis, on the other hand, frequently involves more than one root as depicted in diagram (*D*) where the fourth lumbar nerve root is compressed as it passes through the subarticular gutter and the fifth lumbar nerve root is kinked around the pedicle of L5.

facets to a marked degree. This can be demonstrated on the lateral view by the fact that joint body line—a line drawn along the caudal border of the vertebral body—when extended posteriorly cuts through the middle of the facet instead of passing over the top of it (fig. 10.24). In chronic subluxations the inferior articular fact impinges on the lamina below where a reactive ridge of bone is formed. This reactive ridge of bone is recognizable on clinical radiographs as a white crescent on the oblique view.

In the anteroposterior view, a line drawn along the inferior border of the transverse process over the pars interarticularis and the joint below will form a smooth "S." When subluxation occurs, this line is interrupted (fig. 10.25). In extreme degrees of subluxation, the tip of the superior articular facet can be seen to impinge against the pedicle above (fig. 10.26).

Narrowing of the interlaminar space noted on the anteroposterior view of the spine is a very characteristic feature of apophysial stenosis. The interlaminar space may be encroached upon by overgrowth of the posterior facets, by abnormal configuration of the laminae, by subluxation of the facets, or by osteoarthritis of the posterior joints.

The findings on myelographic examination differ from those seen with disc ruptures. The myelogram does not show the discreet myelographic

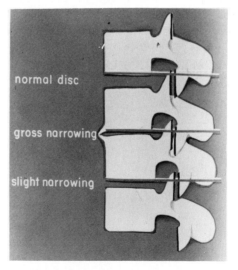

normal disc

gross narrowing

slight narrowing

Fig. 10.24. When an intervertebral disc narrows, the posterior joints must subluxate. This can be demonstrated on the lateral x-ray by drawing a line along the caudal border of a vertebral body and extending it posteriorly (the joint body line). Normally this line passes over the tip of the superior articular facet. If the posterior joints are subluxated, then this line cuts through the middle of the facet.

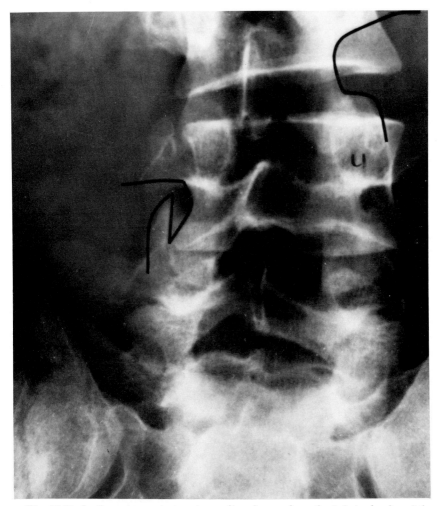

Fig. 10.25. In the anteroposterior view, a line drawn along the inferior border of the transverse process over the pars interarticularis and the joint below will form a smooth "S." When subluxation occurs, this line is interrupted. In this x-ray this phenomenon is depicted at the L4-L5 joint on the right.

defect commonly seen with a rupture of an intervertebral disc. There may be root sleeve cut-off, either unilaterally or bilaterally, and commonly there may be waisting of the oil column. This latter myelographic finding is of importance because it may be erroneously interpreted as representing a "central disc rupture." Degenerative spinal stenosis is frequently associated with a diffuse annular bulge. The posterior hump produced by the diffuse annular bulge as it intrudes into

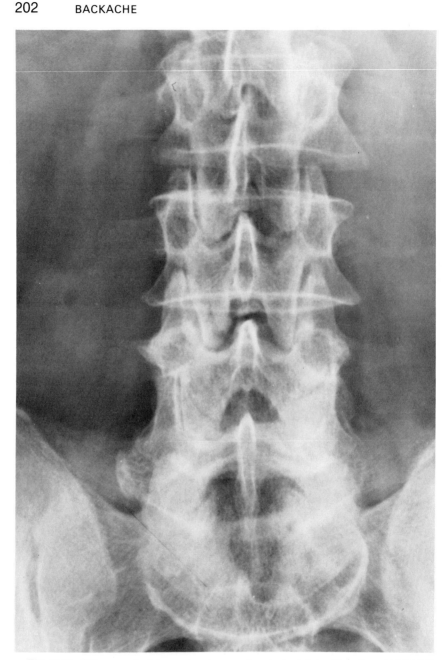

Fig. 10.26. This x-ray depicts varying degrees of posterior joint subluxation. At L2-L3 it can be seen that the tip of the superior articular facet of L3 is about 1 cm distal to the transverse process of L2. At the L3-L4 segment, the tip of the superior articular facet almost touches the pedicle above. At the L4-L5 segment the tip of the superior articular facet of L5 abuts against the pedicle and base of the transverse process of L4. This is particularly noticeable on the right.

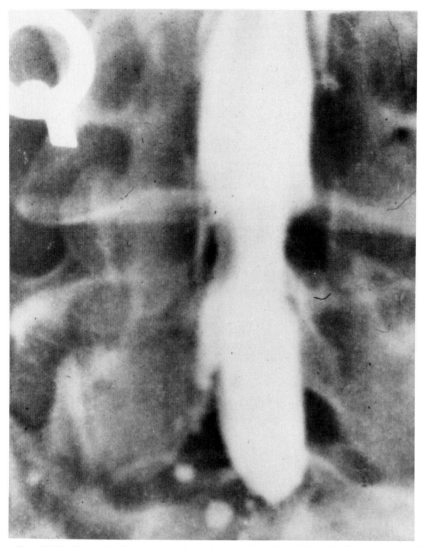

Fig. 10.27. The typical waisting or hourglass constriction of the oil column associated with a diffuse annular bulge, commonly seen with degenerative segmental stenosis.

the spinal canal produces a watershed effect, and as the dye in the subarachnoid space hurries over this eminence, the increased rate of flow is associated with narrowing of the oil column producing a waisting or hourglass constriction at this segment (fig. 10.27).

If the bony constriction is confined to the apophysial area, the myelogram may be normal. If the myelogram is normal and the x-rays show a very narrow disc corresponding to the root involved, the clinician can be certain that the patient is suffering from compression of the nerve root in the foramen at this level.

When lateral encroachment is combined with laminar constriction of the spinal canal, with or without a diffuse bulge of the annulus, there may be a complete cut-off in the flow of dye. The paint brush or rat tail appearance at the end of the oil column distinguishes this myelographic defect from that produced by a tumor which shows a characteristic and pathognomonic meniscus.

Laminar compression of the posterior aspect of the cauda equina is revealed on myelography by segmentation of the oil column at one or more levels. The fact that the compression is posterior is shown on the lateral view.

In the bony root entrapment syndromes, then, the myelograms are difficult to interpret. When the clinical findings are equivocal and the myelogram does not reveal the level of the lesion, it is frequently necessary to determine the level of root involvement by root sleeve infiltration and by electromyography.

The indications for surgical intervention are the same as those for any patient with root compromise, namely, persisting disabling symptoms resisting all forms of conservative therapy or else evidence of severe or increasing root involvement.

If the patient's symptoms become severe enough to demand complete bedrest, the prognosis of conservative therapy, by prolonging bedrest, is not so good as the prognosis of a patient suffering from a disc herniation. This is understandable. A disc herniation may resolve and the protrusion recede with the fibrotic reaction of healing. All that can be achieved by bedrest for a patient suffering from root compromise due to a bony entrapment is the hope that the inflammatory reaction around the root will subside, and that when the root has decreased in size it will lie at ease despite the narrowing of the root canal. It is advisable, therefore, that conservative therapy should include the use of anti-inflammatory drugs given systemically. If these fail to produce any significant improvement, steroids may be given epidurally or by root sleeve infiltration.

In summary, then, the most important feature of spinal stenosis is the recognition of this pathological entity as a source of back and leg pain, particularly in the older age group. It must be remembered that the symptoms may be produced by compression of the dura by the lamina, by bony compression of the emerging nerve roots, or by a combination of these two mechanisms at the same level or at different levels. The only hope of conservative therapy is to reduce the inflammatory response in the involved nerve root.

Because of this, anti-inflammatory medication should be employed.

If the patient fails to improve on conservative therapy and remains significantly disabled, surgical decompression must be considered.

In the preoperative evaluation of these patients, it is important to attempt to localize the level of nerve root involvement accurately by clinical evaluation, reinforced by myelography, and, if the findings on myelography are equivocal, further ancillary investigations must be carried out, including electromyography and nerve root infiltration.

The significance of laminar compression revealed on myelography must be assessed in the light of the clinical picture and the extent of the required decompression designed accordingly, either apophysial or laminar decompression or a combination of both.

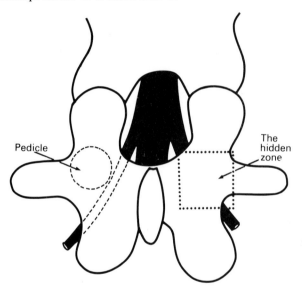

Fig. 10.28. The hidden zone.

Table 10.3. Features Differentiating Disc Ruptures from Root Entrapment by Bony Overgrowth

Clinical Picture	Disc Rupture	Bony Root Entrapment
Age	Under 40	Over 50
Backache	Short duration	Long duration
Straight leg raising	Limited	Not limited
No. of segments	One	Several
Significant x-ray changes	None	Several
Myelographic defects	Common	May be normal
	Unilateral	Bilateral
	Anterior	Posterior

Table 10.4. Causes of Sciatic Pain

A. Thalamic pain
B. Radicular pain
   1. Arteriovenous malformation
   2. Nerve root tumors and cysts
   3. Extradural root compression
      a. Disc ruptures
      b. Bony entrapment
      c. Periradicular fibrosis
      d. Hematoma
      e. Vertebral abscess
      f. Vertebral neoplasm
C. Lesion of sciatic plexus
   1. Direct trauma (forceps delivery)
   2. Pelvic infections
   3. Endometriosis
   4. Pelvic neoplasms
   5. Sacroiliac joint lesions
      a. Inflammations—sacroiliitis
      b. Infections—pyogenic, tuberculous
      c. Trauma
D. Sciatic nerve
   1. Contusions
   2. Neoplasms
   3. Neuritides
      a. Toxic
      b. Infective
      c. Viral
      d. Metabolic
E. Referred pain
   1. Disc degeneration
   2. Sacroiliac joint lesions
   3. Arthritis of hip joint
   4. Ischial bursitis
   5. Cyst of lateral cartilage of knee
   6. Baker's cyst
   7. Lesions of femur
      a. Infections
      b. Neoplasms
      c. Paget's disease
F. Vascular
   1. Tibial compartmental syndromes
   2. Peripheral vascular disease

If the true nature of the underlying pathology has been missed in the preoperative evaluation and the source of root compression erroneously attributed to a disc herniation, at operation it will be found that the nerve root is still tight after removal of the disc material and cannot be displaced medially. Under such circumstances the root is tethered in the hidden zone and must be followed to its point of emergence, if necessary, to find the source and cause of root fixation (fig. 10.28).

The clinical features differentiating a bony root entrapment from a disc rupture are summarized in table 10.3.

Only two sources of sciatic pain have been described in detail: referred pain secondary to degenerative disc disease and the root compression syndromes. Sciatic pain may occur as a result of a toxic or infective neuritis; it may be referred from lesions outside the spine such as a trochanteric bursitis or a cyst of the lateral cartilage of the knee; it may be derived from intrapelvic lesions giving rise to irritation of the sciatic plexus; or it may be due to compression or irritation of the sciatic nerve itself throughout its course. the possible causes of the subjective complaint of "sciatica" are summarized in table 10.4.

CHAPTER 11

Failures of Spinal Surgery

"Look! In this place, ran Cassius dagger through:
See, what a rent the envious Casca made:
Through this, the well behaved Brutus stabbed."
—William Shakespeare

"There is not a fiercer hell than the failure in a great object."
—John Keats

One of the most difficult problems of orthopedic surgery is the assessment and management of patients still seriously disabled by backache, despite one or more attempts at surgical correction of the underlying lesion. Such failures are nearly always compounded by a variable and varying mixture of inadequate preoperative assessments, errors in operative technique, and emotional breakdown of the patient either antedating or following surgery. It is convenient to consider these separately under the headings of failure following discectomy; failure following laminectomy for spinal stenosis; failure of spinal fusion; and persistent symptoms in the emotionally destroyed.

FAILURES FOLLOWING DISCECTOMY

No Relief of Sciatic Pain

If the patient gives the history that following laminectomy there was no change in the degree of leg pain, the first possibility that has to be considered is that the preoperative diagnosis was erroneous. The patient may have been suffering from referred pain and not root irritation, and there is no way that a laminectomy can relieve the symptoms of pain referred from an unstable spinal segment.

The wrong level may have been explored.

Probably one of the most common causes of failure is the lack of recognition of the bony root entrapment syndromes, particularly if preoperatively the myelogram appears to show a defect interpreted as a "central disc." At operation this diffusely bulging annulus may be

208

recognized and erroneously felt to be the source of the patient's sciatic pain. If the nerve root, however, was in reality compressed as it coursed through the subarticular gutter, then obviously removal of the disc, even though it was bulging, would not relieve the patient's pain.

Persistence of sciatic pain following a laminectomy for a disc herniation associated with an anomaly of root emergence is a distressing phenomenon. It would appear, particularly in those examples in which there are two nerve roots emerging through the same foramen, that the conjoined nerve roots become edematous as a result of the disc herniation and thereby are subjected to a further constraint within the foramen. Following the discectomy the root swelling persists and the foraminal entrapment likewise persists. It would appear wise in the presence of this type of root anomaly always to combine a discectomy with a foraminotomy, allowing the nerve root to lie completely free up to its point of emergence.

The continuing sciatic pain may have been due to an error in technique, such as incomplete removal of nuclear material with subsequent extrusion of more nucleus in the immediate postoperative period. A sequestrated fragment may have been overlooked, particularly if this has migrated down the foramen. This error will be obviated if, at the conclusion of every laminectomy, the surgeon takes special care to look underneath the dura and follow the nerve root to its point of emergence with a blunt probe.

The surgeon must never forget that the nerve root will find a textile foreign body a very irritating companion. It is wise to make sure that these useful handmaidens of surgical technique are radiopaque.

Recurrence of Sciatic Pain

If the patient states that following laminectomy the sciatic pain was relieved but subsequently recurred, three possibilities must be borne in mind: a recurrent disc rupture at the same level or more commonly at another level; bony root compression resulting from disc collapse; and the development, postoperatively, of peridural and/or periradicular fibrosis.

This fibrotic response will give rise to a slowly progressive recurrence of sciatic pain. The amount of scarring produced appears to be proportional to the size of the laminotomy defect and the amount of epidural hematoma. The scar may spread, on occasion, all around the dura, around the nerve roots and out into the intervertebral foramina. The periradicular scar may mat the nerve root densely to the back of the disc, with the rootlets showing an almost malignantly invasive intraneural fibrosis. This fibrotic response is dependent solely on the operative exposure which must always be kept in mind when considering re-exploration following laminectomy, because the second exposure will be large and further peridural fibrosis will occur almost inevitably.

Continuing Disabling Backache

Following discectomy the sciatic pain may be relieved, but the patient may be plagued by continuing back pain. In many of these patients, if you go back over their initial history you will find that their story was one of recurrent episodes of backache of increasing severity, duration, and frequency, culminating in an attack of incapacitating sciatic pain which necessitated operative intervention. These patients have been suffering for a long period of time from segmental instability giving rise to low back pain. The disc rupture, even though it precipitated the operative intervention, is only one part of the mechanical insufficiency of the spine. Removal of the disc alone in these patients will leave them with the same type of back pain from which they were complaining in the past. This is the group of patients who should be treated initially by combining discectomy with fusion, where this is feasible.

If the laminectomy involves destruction of the posterior joints, it may well lead to subsequent back pain, particularly if the involved segment is very mobile; indeed, if decompression requires a total excision of one or both posterior joints, then a segmental fusion is mandatory.

FAILURE FOLLOWING LAMINECTOMY FOR SPINAL STENOSIS

Incomplete Apophysial Decompression

Incomplete decompression of the involved nerve roots is seen in the following circumstances.

Entrapment of a Nerve Root at More Than One Site

This error will be avoided if the mobility of the root is assessed after the apparent source of compression is removed (fig. 11.1). It should be possible to displace a normal nerve root at least 1 cm medially.

Involvement of More Than One Root

Incomplete decompression may result when more than one root is involved in an apparently unisegmental degenerative stenosis (fig. 11.2). This source of failure emphasizes the need for complete preoperative evaluation of the roots involved. The surgeon must know what roots to explore.

Overlooked Apophysial Stenosis

A decompression laminectomy for spinal stenosis is always started by the removal of a portion or the whole of one or more laminae. If this is

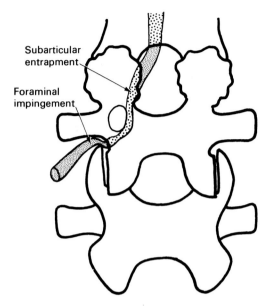

Fig. 11.1. The emerging nerve root may be compressed at more than one site. In this diagram, the nerve root is shown to be compressed as it passes through the subarticular gutter. It is also trapped in the foramen by the tip of the superior articular facet.

technically difficult because of shingling or overgrowth of the laminae, it is understandable that the surgeon confine his attention to a midline decompression, until such time as pulsation is restored to the cauda equina, particularly if the myelogram has revealed a startling segmentation of the oil column. Even though a very complete midline decompression is performed, the patient will not be helped if, as is commonly the case, he is suffering from both laminar stenosis and concomitant apophysial stenosis giving rise to root compression (fig. 11.3). This error is more likely to occur if the apophysial stenosis is at a different segment from the laminar stenosis.

Here again an accurate preoperative assessment followed by a preoperative design of the procedure required will avoid this only too frequent source of error.

Incomplete Midline Decompression

Sometimes a midline decompression is incomplete. It is to be remembered that this operation is most frequently performed on older patients with the surgeon being understandably reluctant to carry out extensive surgery. The operation is frequently tedious, hemorrhagic, time-consuming, and apparently destructive. Despite the temptation to short-circuit the operative procedure, when the patient's symptoms

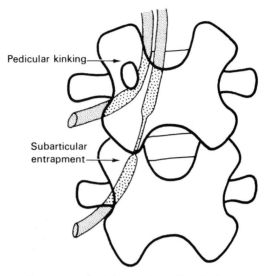

Fig. 11.2. Diagram showing apophysial stenosis resulting in the compression of two nerve roots.

superficially appear to stem from laminar compression at one or two segments only, decompression must be continued until the dura is seen to pulsate once again and epidural fat is seen.

Persisting Backache

As in a laminectomy carried out for a simple disc herniation, if the posterior joints are destroyed, instability invariably arises which may give rise to significant back pain. On occasion, an iatrogenic spondylolisthesis with forward displacement of the involved vertebra is seen in the postoperative period. If decompression necessitates ablation of the posterior joints, the involved segments should be stabilized by an intertransverse fusion.

Peridural Fibrosis

As mentioned previously when the complications of a simple laminectomy for removal of a disc were discussed, one of the problems that may arise is subsequent peridural and periradicular fibrosis. This unfortunate sequel is much more likely to occur in the extensive laminectomy required for decompression of the cauda equina and the emerging nerve roots in a patient suffering from multisegmental spinal stenosis. At the conclusion of the laminectomy, therefore, an interposition membrane should be placed between the dura and the sacrospinales. The best biological membrane presently available is the deepest layer of the dermis. This can be used to reconstitute the ligamentum flavum.

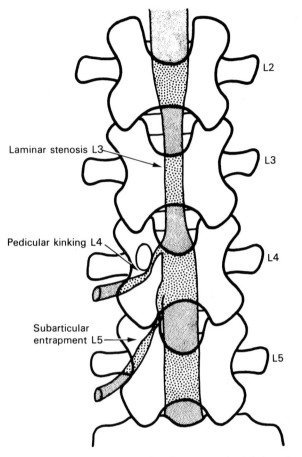

Fig. 11.3. Diagram to show root compression due to apophysial stenosis occurring at different segments from the midline or laminar stenosis.

Preoperative Evaluation

When undertaking the surgical management of patients with continuing or recurrent sciatic pain, it is imperative to localize the involved root accurately prior to operation. This may, at times, be extremely difficult. It is difficult to determine whether the clinical signs of impairment of root conduction are new or whether they are stigmata of a previous episode of root compression.

The ankle jerk, for example, will rarely return to normal after it has been lost. Sensory recovery may be incomplete, and motor power itself may not fully recover.

Myelograms are usually difficult to interpret because the deformation of the oil column may result from peridural fibrosis. Similarly, lack of filling of the internal vertebral veins on selective lumbar phlebography may also be due to the postoperative scarring.

Probably the most useful ancillary investigation is nerve root infiltration. On occasion, particularly at the lumbosacral disc where infiltration of the first sacral root may prove to be technically difficult, a diagnostic discography or discometric analysis of the disc may prove to be of great localizing value if on injecting the lumbosacral disc the clinically experienced symptoms are reproduced.

Because decompression may well involve facetectomy and this in turn necessitates segmental stabilization, it is wiser, preoperatively, to assess the state of health of the discs above the proposed site of exploration, by discography, so that the extent of any fusion required can be accurately defined before operation is undertaken.

FAILURES FOLLOWING SPINAL FUSION

Failures following spinal fusion may be considered under the headings of pain derived from the grafted area, pain derived from the spine above the graft, donor site pain, scar tissue pain due to water logging, or a totally independent spinal lesion.

Pain Derived from the Grafted Areas

Pseudarthrosis

Radiologically a pseudarthrosis may be difficult to demonstrate. Moreover, a pseudarthrosis can be present without pain and the mere demonstration of the lesion does not necessarily mean that the source of the patient's continuing disability has been found.

Increasing work tolerance following infiltration of the pseudarthrosis with local anesthetic tends to indict the lesion as the source of pain, although it must be remembered that an injection of this nature is a powerful hypnotic suggestion. In order to arrive at any valid conclusion, it is necessary to assess the suggestibility of the patient first by observing the result of injection of normal saline.

Discography may well prove to be the best diagnostic tool. Discography in the presence of a solid fusion, although demonstrating an irregular pattern, is generally painless. If there is a pseudarthrosis, discography is painful at the involved segment. This technique carries with it an accuracy rate of about 80%.

In the surgical management of a pseudarthrosis, the failure rate of refusion has been alarmingly high. This probably arises from the fact that it is difficult to obtain, in the fusion area, a good vascular bed with a potent source of osteoblasts capable of revascularizing and reossifying the graft. It is best to reoperate on the spine in an area in which there has been no previous interference.

If the previous fusion was midline, an intertransverse fusion is the best approach for repair. If the previous fusion was intertransverse, then the fusion bed should be along the spinous processes. If the previous fusion was a combination of an intertransverse and posterior fusion, the so-called "Cowl" fusion, then an anterior interbody fusion is the only feasible method of salvage.

Root Compression

The patient may develop symptoms and signs of root compression which may be due to a rupture of an intervertebral disc underneath the fusion or it may be due to an iatrogenic spinal stenosis. A ruptured disc very rarely occurs under a solid spinal fusion; it is much more likely to occur in the presence of a pseudarthrosis. In those instances in which there is a ruptured disc under a fusion which is irrefutably solid, in all probability it was present at the time the fusion was performed.

Whereas the symptoms resulting from a recent disc rupture are fairly rapid in onset, the symptoms resulting from an iatrogenic spinal stenosis are *slow* in developing (fig. 11.4). The clinical picture is clear-cut. A patient with a solid spinal fusion, usually midline and incorporating the

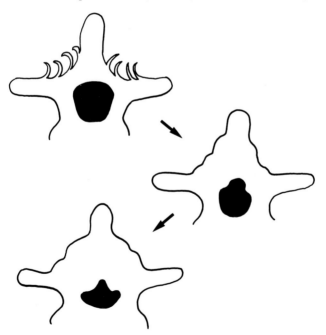

Fig. 11.4. Any operative procedure that involves decortication of the lamina may result subsequently in gross thickening of the lamina. If the spinal canal was narrow at the time of operation, further narrowing induced by the thickening of the lamina may precipitate the symptoms of spinal stenosis.

L4-L5 segment, which prior to operation had radiological evidence of interlaminar narrowing, slowly develops the claudicant type of sciatic pain that one associates with root compression secondary to spinal stenosis. On examination, these patients frequently present evidence of impairment of root conduction at more than one segment.

Pain Derived from the Spine above the Graft

Spondylolysis Acquisita

A spondylolysis may develop at the segment above the spinal fusion. Spondylolysis acquisita is probably much more common than previously acknowledged because it may well be missed on a routine lateral view taken for the postoperative assessment of the stability of a spinal fusion. It is probably advisable in all patients who have undergone a spinal fusion and subsequently suffer from persisting discomfort to take oblique views of the spine to show the pars interarticularis of the segment above the lesion.

The exact etiology of the lesion is not known. It may be a stress fracture. The development of a stress fracture may be predisposed to by dissection of the muscle masses away from the lamina at the segment above a spinal fusion. A dissection such as this would interfere to a fairly marked degree with the venous drainage of the lamina, giving rise to partial death of bone in this area. If subsequently extra stresses are placed on such a bone by the placement of a graft below it, then the pars interarticularis may break and spondylolysis develop.

The lesion is not seen in patients in whom an intertransverse fusion has been carried out. Theoretically, spondylolysis acquista should not occur with an intertransverse fusion because the site of the lesion is supported by the uppermost portion of the graft (fig. 11.5).

Lumbodorsal Strain

The significance of a chronic lumbodorsal strain following a lumbosacral fusion has not been sufficiently recognized. When the lumbosacral segment is fused, extra mechanical stresses are placed on the lumbodorsal junction and a previously asymptomatic degenerative change at this level may, following lumbosacral fusion, produce pain referred to both buttocks and down as low as the great trochanters.

Here again, treatment is prophylactic, recognizing the possibility and investigating the probability in every patient considered for spinal fusion. If the lesion does occur, there is no reason why a localized segmental fusion should not be undertaken.

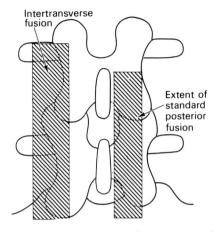

Fig. 11.5. An intertransverse fusion supports the pars interarticularis of the proximal vertebral segment in a spinal fusion. Because of this, spondylolysis acquisita is not seen with intertransverse fusions.

Donor Site Pain

Continuing pain may be derived from the donor site. The superficial gluteal nerve crosses the iliac crest about four fingers' breadth away from the midline (fig. 11.6). If an incision over the iliac crest is used to obtain the graft, the superficial gluteal nerve may be divided and trapped in the scar and become a source of pain. It is preferable to curve the lower end of the midline incision to expose the posterior superior iliac spine and obtain bone from this site.

In those instances in which a gluteal neuroma develops, the tenderness is exquisitely well localized and the pain can be temporarily abolished by infiltration of the area with local anesthetic. Under such circumstances it is worthwhile to explore the incision and look for the neuroma. When it is found, the stump of the gluteal nerve should be caught in forceps and pulled as hard as possible to deliver the nerve into the wound to permit division of the nerve 2 inches proximal to the point where it crosses the iliac crest.

Sacroiliac Pain

Sacroiliac instability may occur if the donor site encroaches markedly on the sacroiliac joint, particularly if the iliolumbar ligament is divided. This is probably the most important of all the stabilizing ligaments of the sacroiliac joint. In cadavers, if this ligament is divided, the sacroiliac joint can be opened up easily, like the two halves of a book.

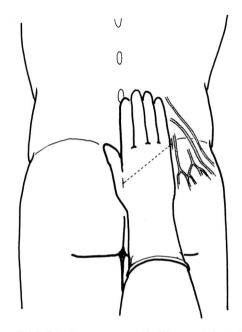

Fig. 11.6. The superficial gluteal nerve crosses the iliac crest about four fingers' breadth away from the midline.

Patients with sacroiliac instability will present with pain over the sacroiliac joint and the pain will radiate down the lateral aspect of the great trochanter onto the front of the thigh. Weight bearing on the involved extremity increases the pain and the patients tend to limp with a combined Trendelenburg and antalgic gait. The pain is reproduced by straining the sacroiliac joints by resisted abduction of the hip and is temporarily relieved by infiltration of the involved sacroiliac joint with local anesthetic. With gross instability, movement at the symphysis pubis may be observed when the x-rays are taken with the patient standing first on one leg, then on the other (fig. 11.7).

Some of these patients may even require a sacroiliac fusion to get rid of this troublesome, residual, significant disability.

Scar Tissue Pain

One has to accept the fact that scar tissue itself may be a source of pain. If extensive scarring occurs because of a postoperative hematoma or a low grade infection, it is difficult with loss of the pumping effect of muscle action to obtain adequate tissue fluid drainage and the scar becomes water-logged. As in any other tissue, distension by fluid accumulation gives rise to a dull, constant boring discomfort. Muscle

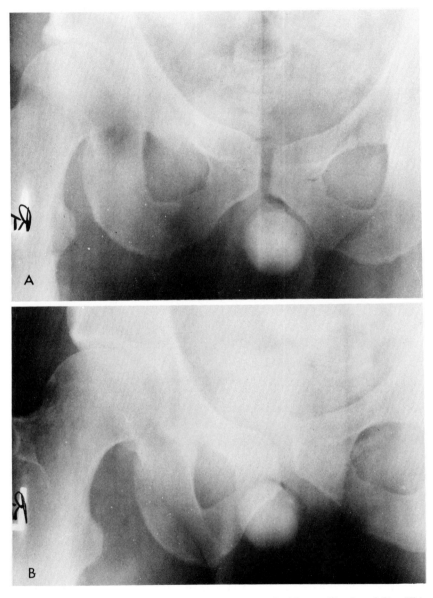

Fig. 11.7. Instability of the symphysis pubis associated with sacroiliac instability. This patient had instability of the left sacroiliac joint. In the first x-ray (A) the patient is standing on his right leg, and in the second x-ray (B) he is taking full weight on his left leg. Note the gross excursion of the symphysis pubis that is demonstrated when the patient takes his weight on the left leg.

retraining may be of some value. To enable the patient to build up muscle tone by increased activities, it may be necessary to employ neuromodulation of pain by percutaneous electrical stimulation. This decreases the discomfort temporarily and permits increased activities which, in turn, encourage the pumping action of the sacrospinales.

Miscellaneous Causes

It must be remembered that the performance of a spinal fusion does not protect the patient against other forms of spinal diseases such as tuberculosis, secondary deposits, etc. The physician must be wary lest the history of a previous assault on the spine focus his attention too rigidly on some small portion of the back, with the result that he ignores, or overlooks, gross pathology at another level.

PERSISTENT SYMPTOMS IN THE EMOTIONALLY DESTROYED PATIENT

When assessing why a patient is still disabled following surgical intervention, it is vitally important to assess the patient as a whole. The clinician must go right back to the beginning of the sad story. He must learn of the onset of the pain, its character, and the degree of disability developing which necessitated eventual surgical intervention. He must, in retrospect, once again reassess this disability and determine whether it was indeed within the bounds of reason.

Only too frequently, prior to the initial surgery, the surgeon is faced with a patient who has a protracted disability. He has been in and out of work; he has been in and out of hospital; he has been in and out of physical therapy departments; and he has been in and out of the offices of drugless practitioners. It is understandably tempting to regard this long period of disability as indicating severe pain. However, if this group of patients, suffering from low back pain only, cannot be retrained to undertake lighter jobs, then a desperation fusion will be unlikely to succeed.

In this regard it must be emphasized that a patient cannot describe his pain; he can only describe his disability. Pain and disability are not synonymous and the disability complained of is not necessarily indicative of the degree of pain experienced.

In the simplest superficial analysis, disability has two components: the pain and the patient's reaction to the pain. A certain degree of what might be termed a functional reaction can be regarded as normal. When the functional response is gross, it becomes a major part of the disease process. This concept is best exemplified by describing three hypothetical workmen, three bricklayers who presented with the same degree of disability. They had pain in their backs; although they could walk around, they could not do their work. They could not climb ladders. They could not carry bricks. They could not stoop to lay the bricks. They were not able to describe the amount of pain they had; they could only describe their disability. They all had degenerative disc disease. The x-rays could not describe how much pain they were experiencing. Discograms revealed symptomatic levels which were the same in each patient, but the discograms could not assess the amount of pain produced. All that was known was that the disability claimed by all three was the same: they could not work. In one patient (patient A) the disability was largely due to the anatomical basis of his pain. In another patient (patient C) there was little anatomical source of pain, but he was overcome by the functional reaction or the emotional response to his discomforts (fig. 11.8).

Surgery meticulously performed might overcome 90% of the anatomical basis of the disability. The first patient (A) would be cured and would be able to return to work, but even with 90% of the organic basis of his disability removed, the third patient (C) would still be incapacitated (fig. 11.9). In such instances, because of failure of treatment, the functional reaction will get worse and the story of patient C is best exemplified by the letters that were written to the Workmen's Compensation Board about him:

"Dear Sirs:

I saw this very pleasant claimant, George Smith, today and the poor fellow has not responded to conservative therapy at all. He is totally unable to work. His x-rays show marked disc degeneration and I plan to bring him into hospital for a local fusion."

"Dear Sirs:

I operated on George today and I am sure he will do well."

"Dear Sirs:

I saw George Smith today and I am a little disappointed with his progress to date."

"Dear Sirs:

Smith's x-rays show a solid fusion, but he shows surprisingly little motivation to return to work."

"Dear Sirs:

This dreadful fellow Smith."

"Dear Sirs:

Smith obviously needs psychiatric help" (fig. 11.10).

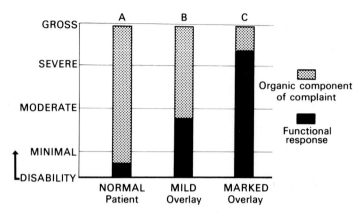

Fig. 11.8. Functional overlay. Three patients (A, B, and C) with apparently identical disability.

Patient A, patient B, and patient C all presented with the same disability. They were bricklayers who could not work. They had the same x-ray changes, they had similar discograms, but the constitution of their disability varied enormously and, predictably, the results of operative treatment varied also (fig. 11.11).

In patient C, the degenerative disc disease was not causing too much pain, and in better emotional health, the discomfort he experienced would not have taken him to a doctor. However, because of factors outside his spine, in fact outside his soma, he was totally disabled by this discomfort; and this disability was later compounded, perpetuated, and exaggerated by the failure of surgical treatment.

Patient A and patient C do not really constitute much of a problem because the gross functional overlay of patient C is usually recognizable. These two groups of patients have been discussed in detail to emphasize the fact that pain and disability are not synonymous.

The middle group, patient B, typifies the most commonly seen problem. The surgeon who regards a functional overlay as a solid contraindication to operation will not help patient B because he does have an organic basis of discomfort.

There are two important aspects in the mangement of these patients that must always be borne in mind: first, the recognition of the organic basis of pain, despite the clouding of the clinical picture by the functional elements; and second, an analysis of the constitution of the functional component of the disability.

The functional overlay is derived from a combination of many factors. A large part of the emotional overlay is due to the patient's personality; he may have no drive, no motivation, he may even be a psychopath.

Whatever it is, it probably cannot be altered. It is important to recognize a gross personality defect because these patients won't do well with treatment directed solely at their spine.

Other factors must be considered, such as the patient's affect or mood, the significance of pain to the patient, and the patient's ability to adjust to his environment. The importance of financial security and work demands are obvious. Finally, the reaction of the patient to pain must be considered: his pain tolerance and his pain threshold. If the patient, because of inheritance or constitution, for example, tends to have an exaggerated reaction to any painful stimulus, it makes it very difficult to recognize the fact that the patient is suffering from an organic lesion.

For example, a patient may react violently at the limit of one phase of clinical examination: straight leg raising. On experiencing discomfort, he

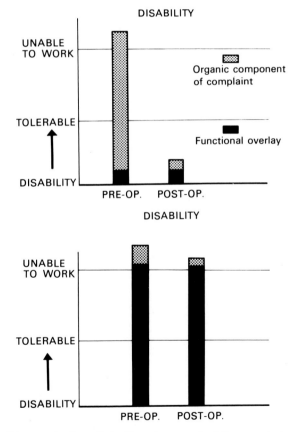

Fig. 11.9. Diagram to show that although removal of the organic basis of pain will produce a good result in the emotionally stable patient A (*top*), the continuing emotional turmoils in patient C (*bottom*) result in perpetuation of his disability following operation.

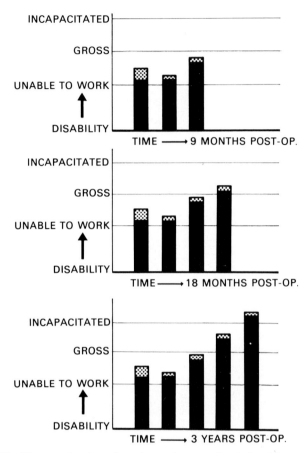

Fig. 11.10. Diagram to show how increasing emotional breakdown will produce increasing disability following surgical intervention.

may writhe, groan, shout, bang his hands, and finally collapse, sobbing and weeping. Such patients react excessively to pain produced by an organic disability. However, when this excessive reaction is of a hysterical nature, it becomes extremely difficult to determine whether the problem is one of a hysterical patient with pain or a patient with hysterical pain.

It is very important to differentiate two types of emotional response: one is the psychogenic regional pain syndrome in which there is no underlying organic basis for the patient's complaints which represent one facet of a significant emotional breakdown, and the other is a disability arising from a gross psychogenic magnification of symptoms derived from a relatively minor underlying physical disorder.

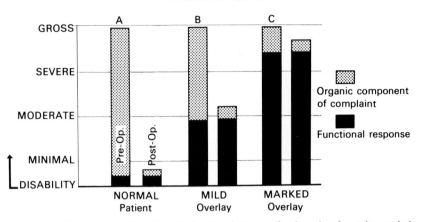

Fig. 11.11. Diagram to show the relationship between the functional overlay and the response to treatment in patients A, B, and C.

Psychogenic Regional Pain

Allan Walters described psychogenic regional pain as "a class of functional pain for which the clinician can find no clinical cause and which is often called 'hysterical' or simply 'psychogenic.'" These pains which are evoked without any peripheral excitation occur not only in hysteria, but throughout the whole range of neuroses, psychoses, situational states, and minor reactions to everyday life. These pains have a regional distribution which is their hallmark. The regions are topographical units variously innervated. This is completely different from the physiogenic pain pattern of scattered sites of pain having a common innervation.

Steindler stated, "It is dangerous to arrogate to oneself the opinion that what one cannot explain does not exist."

This observation is particularly applicable to the diagnosis of psychogenic pain. It is unsafe to presume that a pain must be based on some pathological change just because the patient appears to be emotionally stable, and it is equally unsafe to conclude that the pain is psychogenically induced just because no obvious abnormality can be found. The diagnosis of psychogenic regional pain is a positive diagnosis, dependent on positive findings. It is not a diagnosis arrived at by exclusion by failing to find any obvious pathological lesion. The following positive physical findings should be noted on examination.

Skin Tenderness

Tenderness evoked by just lightly touching the skin or pinching it may be noted. The action of pinching the skin in a small area may send pain radiating through the whole region. This phenomenon is only seen in psychogenic regional pain.

Deep Tenderness

If there is skin tenderness, no statement can be made as to the presence of deep tenderness. As Allan Walters stated, "This is a trap for those clinicians whose fingers dip deeply without first reconnoitering the skin."

In the absence of skin tenderness, psychogenic regional deep tenderness is characterized by the presence of contiguous areas of tenderness elicited over large areas not localized to anatomical boundaries of innervation. Characteristically, these patients will present with areas of tenderness over the subcutaneous border of the tibia.

Sensory Deficits

These are the well known areas of stocking or glove "hysterical" anesthesia. Sharp unanatomical boundaries are common, but shaded and patchy marginal zones may occur. Varying and variable zones of anesthesia are common. Commonly the patients demonstrate a zone of hypoesthesia over the site of maximal pain. This is the most characteristic feature of a psychogenic regional pain, and it may be missed if there does not appear to be any reason to carry out a neurological examination.

Motor Weakness

Characteristically, these patients show discrepant motor weakness. They may be able to maintain a posture, for example, dorsiflexion of the ankle, but cannot achieve dorsiflexion from the plantar flexed position against even the slightest force.

Abnormal motor weakness commonly extends beyond the region of pain. The patients may be unable to hold their eyes squeezed tightly shut against the attempts of the examiner to open the eyes gently with his index finger and thumb. Even though their complaint is of back pain, they may have difficulty in extending the terminal interphalangeal joint of their thumb against resistance.

Reflex Changes

It is not commonly recognized that superficial and deep tendon reflexes may be suppressed by psychic factors. Psychogenic areflexia becomes a major diagnostic trap in the psychogenic regional pain syndrome, if the presence of areflexia is taken as irrefutable evidence of anatomical denervation. When areflexia is associated with other regional features, the psychogenic possibility should never be ignored.

Vegatative Changes

Increased or decreased sweating, regional vasoconstriction, or vasodilation and dermatographia may also be present.

The mimicry is so great that the gravest danger of psychogenic regional pain is for the physician to fail to recognize its existence and thereby, on occasion, be misled so far as to advise surgical procedures.

Psychogenic Magnification

Patients with a hysterical personality frequently present with psychogenic magnification of pain. The surgeon, of course, is always treating a patient and not a spine; regardless of the bizarre description of the symptoms or the histrionics on examination, the surgeon must accept the possibility of physical disorder and investigate its probability in every instance. Psychological testing will not reveal how much of the persisting symptoms are due to emotional factors. Admittedly, subjecting a patient to a battery of psychological tests would inform the clinician of the bizarre nature of the patient's emotional constitution, but unfortunately, will not tell the clinician whether this peculiar fellow is suffering from degenerative disc disease or even if he is suffering from a secondary deposit in his spine.

The clinician must listen carefully to the story and the description of the disability. As mentioned previously when emotional overtones were described, a patient whose disability stems from a psychogenic magnification of the symptoms frequently grossly exaggerates the discomforts he experiences, "I get attacks of pain when I am paralyzed and cannot move."

Sometimes the patients find it difficult to describe clear-cut symptoms, and they give the impression of a person struggling to remember a dream. Sometimes the description of pain reveals that is not related in any way to activity.

The variations in the history indicative of emotional overtones are indeed manifold and often, at times, surprisingly deceptive. They never ring entirely true and a clear impression is gained that you are hearing the words of a song without the music. On examination, the patient frequently points to the area of discomfort with his thumb, never actually touching the skin. The patient may present a theatrical display of distress, voluble in describing painful reaction to examination with gross and unreasonable limitation of movements of the spine. Straight leg raising is not relieved by flexion of the knee, and further flexion of the hip with the knee bent aggravates the pain.

It may be difficult to differentiate between a psychogenic regional pain and a gross disability produced by a psychogenic magnification of the symptoms and signs derived from a relatively minor organic disorder. The introduction of the thiopental sodium pain assessment by Walters has been of inestimable value in assessing the significance of emotional states and the production of the disability presented by the patient. The basis of this test lies in the fact that, at the stage of light anesthesia, although the patient is unconscious, he is still capable of demonstrating primitive reactions to pain. The patient is anesthetized with thiopental and then allowed to rouse until the corneal reflex returns. At this stage of anesthesia he will withdraw from pinprick and will grimace when a painful stimulus is applied such as squeezing the tendo Achillis. With the patient maintained at this level of anesthesia, maneuvers that were previously painful on clinical examination are re-evaluated. If, for example, with the knee held extended, the patient grimaces when the leg has been raised just 20°, this finding may be taken as irrefutable evidence of significant root tension regardless of the presence of any associated emotional breakdown. If, on the other hand, at the stage of anesthesia where the patient will withdraw from pinprick, straight leg raising which was only 20° on clinical examination can now be carried out to 90° without any response from the patient, the clinician may safely conclude there is no evidence of root tension and that the patient's disability is due to his emotional reactions rather than to any organic source of pain.

This discussion of the psychogenic component on the disability resulting from a back pain was deliberately included in this chapter on the failures of spinal surgery because, unfortunately, the persistence of pain following surgery is only too frequently the first indication that the surgeon has of the emotional content of the patient's disability.

Lack of recognition of the role played by the patient's emotional profile on the continuing disability may lead to fruitless repetitive surgical assaults on the patient's spine with a relentlessly progressive deterioration in the patient's condition. An accumulation of a few of these tragic results may lead the surgeon to blame the procedure for the failures. "We don't do spinal fusions anymore—they're never successful."

The patients may be blamed as a group. "A spinal fusion should never be performed on compensation cases," a remark that ignores the fact that the same group of patients may do well following open reduction of fractures or following meniscectomy.

We all learn about emotional factors affecting results from the failures of spinal surgery. Having recognized and acknowledged this fact, we must apply this knowledge in our preoperative assessment of patients. If we do this assiduously and carefully, the results of surgery will be much more predictable and the failures less frequently seen.

CHAPTER 12

Epilogue

"To myself I seem to have been only like a boy playing on the sea shore, and diverting myself in now and then finding a smoother pebble or a prettier shell than ordinary, while the great ocean lay all undiscovered before me."

—Sir Isaac Newton

This book has the character of a butterfly, flitting briefly from topic to topic, missing many aspects of back pain and its treatment and never staying long enough to explore any one topic in depth. Its purpose, however, has been to provide a base line philosophy of treatment to which the reader can add from his own personal experiences.

The pain resulting from trauma, infections, metabolic diseases, and tumors has a specific underlying pathology. The clinical syndromes are clearly defined and treatment is along well established lines.

The pain that results from poorly understood mechanical breakdown changes in the intervertebral discs does not have a clear-cut picture. The lack of precise knowledge of the underlying pathology and the exact mechanism of pain production has led to a plethora of vaguely delineated clinical syndromes. Terms such as "facet syndrome," "lumbosacral sprains," "myalgia," "sacroiliac sprain," "spinal arthritis," etc. tell us little more than the fact that the patient is suffering from backache. Even more specific terms such as "disc degeneration" and "disc herniation" are so loosely used as to lose much of their significance. The mechanical picture is further clouded by frequently associated emotional factors that are poorly understood.

I would like to make a plea that we establish a simple nomenclature for the clinical description of the lesions producing low back pain. This must of necessity be extremely simple and broad so that it can be expanded as our knowledge advances.

I would like to conclude this book therefore with a suggested nomenclature of the various low back pain syndromes.

Viscerogenic— Back pain derived from disorders of visceral structures.

Vascular—Back pain and/or sciatic pain derived from changes in the aorta and vessels in the lower extremities.

Table 12.1. Discogenic Back Pain

Disc degeneration ↓ Pedicular kinking	→ Mechanical insufficiency of the spine	Local and/or referred pain	No evidence of root tension
Subarticular entrapment Foraminal encroachment Segmental spinal stenosis	→ Root entrapment	Radicular pain	Minor root tension with or without evidence of impairment of root conduction
Disc rupture	→ Root compression	Radicular pain	Root tension with or without evidence of impairment of root conduction

Neurogenic—Back pain derived from lesions in the central nervous system, spinal cord, and cauda equina excluding extradural compression of emerging nerve roots.

Spondylogenic—Back pain derived from disorders of the spinal column and its associated structures. Spondylogenic back pain can be subclassified as follows:

Osseus:—Pain derived from pathological changes in the bony components of vertebral column and sacroiliac joints: traumatic, inflammatory, infective, neoplastic, metabolic, and, structural (e.g. scoliosis, spondylolisthesis, and spinal stenosis).

Soft Tissue:—Pain derived from traumatic and degenerative changes in muscles, ligaments, and fascia.

Discogenic—Back pain with or without sciatica resulting from structural changes in the intervertebral discs. These can be divided into two major groups:

Disc Degeneration:—Gives rise to back pain with or without *referred* pain to legs, without evidence of nerve root compromise.

Disc Rupture:—Gives rise to radicular pain with or without back pain, always associated with signs of nerve root tension, and occasionally with evidence of impairment of root conduction (table 12.1).

Psychogenic—Two groups of emotional disorders must be recognized when assessing disability in contradistinction to pain.

Psychogenic Regional Pain:—The development of backache and/or sciatica without any underlying pathological disorder.

Psychogenic Magnification of Pain:—Emotionally based exaggeration of pain produced by a pathological disorder, resulting in inappropriate disability.

In the diagnosis and management of a patient presenting with low back pain, the orthopedic surgeon must play many roles: family practitioner, internist, radiologist, physiatrist, orthotist, psychiatrist, social worker, and friend. He should rarely find it necessary to play the role of his chosen avocation—surgeon.

To those of you who have managed to read this book to its last sentence, may I extend my congratulations and gratitude.

INDEX